TALKING ABOUT DYING

In memory of Myfanwy

A beloved wife, mother, teacher and
encourager

Thanks be to God

Philip Giddings has profound and deeply reflected experience of personal loss, and has, with much courage, brought this book together. It offers thoughtful, practical and pastoral advice on matters of death and dying from Elaine Sugden. There are some beautiful and moving stories from people who have faced these profound challenges that affect us all. Philip Giddings, Martin Down and Gareth Tuckwell offer their reflections on the Christian hope of resurrection and eternal life in Jesus Christ.

Most Rev. Justin Welby, Archbishop of Canterbury

To talk well about dying requires courage, wisdom and sensitivity, qualities much in evidence in this timely book. The authors are unafraid to face head-on the realities of death, whether sudden or expected, violent or natural. Particular care is taken in responding to those most difficult of deaths – those of children, and those by suicide. Practical advice merges with real-life storytelling, making this a book to read now, as well as to keep close by, for we know not what tomorrow brings. All is framed within a realistic compassion, founded on the love we find in Jesus. How faith plays out, and what happens when we pray, are helpfully explored, not least when hopes are dashed and a new, unlooked-for future threatens to overwhelm both ourselves and those whom we love. The temptation is to put things off – making a Will, talking about what really matters. Buy and read this book, and so be equipped for the day when the challenge becomes 'talking about dying'.

Dr Jamie Harrison FRCGP
Dr Harrison worked as a GP for over thirty years, and chairs the House of Laity in the Church of England's General Synod.

This invaluable book comes from a combination of hard wrought personal experience and professional expertise. It considers different kinds of death in a clear, practical and pastorally sensitive way that takes into account the fact that people are very different. What matters is helping them think and talk through issues themselves. Whilst respecting different points of view it is written from the standpoint of the authors' own Christian faith. It can be strongly recommended both for personal use and as a talking point with other people.

Rt Rev. Richard Harries, Baron Harries of Pentregarth
and formerly Bishop of Oxford

About a third of John Wesley's sermons were on dying well – I don't think I have ever heard a sermon on that subject, as the Church has tacitly colluded with our culture's discomfort with the subject. This deeply practical and pastoral book will go a long way to reversing that situation and reducing that discomfort. It would be a hugely helpful resource for every pastor and ordinand.

Rev. Dr Michael Lloyd, Principal of Wycliffe Hall, Oxford

This is one of the most practical books I have come across on dying and the importance of talking about it. The compassion, experience and faith of the authors shine through their realistic contributions. I commend it very warmly indeed for the guidance it offers and the hope it provides.

Rt Rev. James Newcome, Bishop of Carlisle,
Church of England spokesperson for health in the House of Lords

Talking about dying is hard. Knowing what to say and how to say it – as well as knowing what not to say – is difficult for most of us. This clear guide offers helpful advice for patients, relatives, friends and carers, or anyone who finds themselves stuck for words or answers to tricky questions. It covers most eventualities: natural death, violent death, still births and others. It is obvious that the four authors have considerable experience – both personal and professionally in dealing with the challenges dealt with here. Each has a strong Christian faith which adds a spiritual theme to their clear practical and wise advice. This book will be especially valuable to those who are Christians and is a useful addition to the current literature on this difficult topic which, whether we like it or not, is something which one day will affect us all.

Dr Bee Wee, Consultant in Palliative Medicine at
Oxford University Hospitals NHS Foundation Trust

Death is hidden under the carpet by most of us today. We badly need also to be aware of the other fact: life after death. As a Muslim believer and as a medical person, I enjoyed what I read and I learned a lot from this informative and educational book. I admired the rich sources of references and websites after each chapter and at the end of the book. I support most of the ideas and proposals mentioned regarding education about death. I also support fully the idea of using prayer for the healing of our sick patients, which is highly recommended in my religious beliefs.

Dr A. Majid Katme (MBBCH, DPM),
Retired Psychiatrist and
former President of the Islamic Medical Association (UK)

TALKING ABOUT DYING
Help in Facing Death and Dying

Philip Giddings, Martin Down,
Elaine Sugden, Gareth Tuckwell

Wilberforce Publications
London

First published in Great Britain in 2017 by
Wilberforce Publications Limited
70 Wimpole Street, London W1G 8AX
Wilberforce Publications Limited is a wholly owned subsidiary
of Christian Concern

ISBN 978-0-9956832-0-4

Printed in Great Britain by Imprint Digital, Exeter
and worldwide by CreateSpace

Contents

PREFACE

In the course of putting this book together, the issues about dying and death became starkly real when my wife Myfanwy, to whose memory the book is dedicated, suddenly and entirely unexpectedly died of a heart attack aged 69. There was no warning, no time to prepare, no opportunity to say goodbye. It was a devastating experience from which I am still recovering as slowly some scar tissue grows; never before has the full force of the expression 'my other half' come home to me.

In the weeks since that awful day, as I have read and revised our texts, I have reflected not only on the irony of having to face up to unexpected death myself but even more on the importance of having thought and talked about death and dying beforehand – albeit not with my wife, a sad and deeply regrettable omission. If there is one lesson from this painful episode, it is that since death is both inevitable and unpredictable, we owe it to ourselves and our loved ones to be prepared. To this end we offer this book.

Philip Giddings
Lent 2016

FOREWORD

If we are expecting an important event to happen we will usually wish to prepare for it. Some of us will start to prepare early and make detailed arrangements for it. Others will leave the preparations to the last minute so that they require a degree of haste which may damage their completeness. How many of us have left applying for a passport for going abroad until it is almost too late? Few of us will make no preparations at all.

This book is about an important event which is certain to happen and urges us to prepare for it. That event is our own death. When will it occur? Where will it occur and in what circumstances? What are the consequences of it? How can I prepare for an event about which at the present time I know so little?

The four authors are Christian people with a wide range of relevant experience on which to draw. They set out the great variety of occurrences that lead up to death from the sudden and unexpected to a long terminal illness. They use the first of these to stress the utility of talking about death now but they go on to give a rich variety of advice about matters that should be covered in addressing all the circumstances in which death may occur.

After all that there is the question of what happens after death. Is death the end and if not what preparation can I make for what follows? That issue is addressed in a way which I consider readers will find frank and helpful whatever their views may be before they read it.

Our inclination when we and our loved ones are enjoying good health is not to consider how our position may change. This book is a courageous and very well informed call to us to take a realistic view from which great benefit could flow.

Lord Mackay of Clashfern

1

WHY AND HOW DO WE NEED TO TALK ABOUT DYING?

Philip Giddings

What could I say? My old school friend Duncan had just rung to tell me the bad news. I knew he had not been particularly well but it was a shock to hear that, after many tests and treatments, the doctors had concluded that he had inoperable liver cancer and only months to live. He was very matter-of-fact but I could not help wondering what he was really thinking, and whether he was prepared for death. Typically, he did not want to discuss it and expressly forbade me to tell the friends we shared since school.

As the months crept by, I wrestled with the question of what to say to Duncan, his wife and our friends. Should we visit him and, if so, for how long? Yes, we did – but briefly. What to say at Christmas – probably his last? How could we support his wife? We were of a generation in which men 'didn't do feelings'. In our society, there continues to be a wall of silence around the subject of death and dying. All kinds of euphemisms are used to avoid the plain truth. Even medical and caring professionals struggle with how to put it. And often the result is that we end up saying nothing at all.

So too often, after the death of a friend or relative, we find ourselves saying, 'I wish I had been able to say or do . . .' We are too easily put off by fear – both our own fears, and the ones we guess would trouble the dying or their relatives. Too often, we take refuge in talking about trivia and banalities because to introduce the subject of death might seem morbid or demoralizing. So often, we collude with the assumption that the best way to deal with this unpleasant reality is to ignore or deny it – hide our anxieties and sorrow in diversions which we hope will numb our pain at the prospect of losing someone we care about.

This book has been written from our shared conviction that silence will not do. We need to talk about dying and death. We need to do that because it is an unavoidable part of human life: death comes to us all; we can try to ignore its coming, but sooner or later it comes. And before we face our own death, most of us have to deal with the pain of the death of someone close to us – the brute fact of separation from that person. We cannot avoid the fact that our own life, and the lives of those close to us, come to an end.

We also need to talk about dying and death because talking about it will often be helpful to the dying person and their relatives and friends. This is especially so if, as is often the case, talking leads to action on our part or the part of others. We should not lightly avoid the opportunity to show care and love, in word and deed, when we can. 'Talk about' means of course listening as well as speaking and even sharing silence together. Many of us find it difficult to find the words to share our deepest emotions, and that is when an arm round the shoulder or squeeze of the hand speaks more eloquently than mere words.

There are also practical benefits from talking about the approach of death rather than pretending it is not going to happen. There are preparations which need to be made, such as making or updating a will, planning the funeral, making contact with folk with whom one has lost touch, perhaps taking the steps necessary to heal a long-standing breach with a relative, friend or neighbour. Some discussion of these and other matters can help us, and the dying person's relatives and friends, to deal more positively with the death itself and its aftermath.

Yes, but how? What can we say? It is one thing to feel, as I did when Duncan rang, that we ought to talk about dying and death. It is quite another to know how to go about it. As we have discovered whilst preparing to write this book, many people want to talk about death and dying, particularly to close relatives and friends – but do not quite know how. So it is to help them that we have produced this book. Let death no longer be the great unmentionable, but something that we talk about honestly and constructively.

We begin in chapter 2 by looking at the different ways in which people respond to life-threatening illness. Surprising as it may seem, for some, life is enhanced by such an illness as they discover and cherish the people and experiences that really matter to them. By contrast, as we shall see later in chapter 10, some are paralysed by the uncertainty and fear which such an illness brings, even to the extent of refusing to accept what seems inevitable. Whatever our response, there will be difficult decisions to be discussed and taken, especially by those nearest and dearest to the dying person.

In most cases, discussion begins with a conversation with a doctor or consultant about the diagnosis of the illness and how to treat or manage it. Many people find such discussions difficult. So in chapter 3 we consider how we go about talking to doctors and other practitioners about medical decisions. There is a risk that we push doctors into playing the role of God, as patients and relatives want neither to stop treatment nor to take away hope of recovery. In particular, hope is at a premium and too easily it is all focused on the doctor. 'Surely there is something you can do.' Difficult questions can arise at any point of the treatment process: the response to an initial diagnosis of terminal illness; ongoing issues with treatment, curative or palliative; or decisions about withdrawing treatment which is no longer helpful, or not attempting resuscitation. Here we also deal with 'advanced directives' (also known as 'living wills').

A recurrent theme throughout this book is that, like most human beings, we lack control over the circumstances of our own death. We don't know *when* we will die, since mortal disease can often involve significant pain. We may therefore face pressure to shorten that period of pain in various ways, such as by ceasing treatment. We deal with this in chapter 3. Neither do we know *where* we will die – in hospital where medical expertise is at hand or in the more familiar surroundings of one's home, or *how* we will die – and this has been central to the debate on the controversial questions of euthanasia and physician-assisted suicide. In chapter 4, we tackle these difficult questions of when, where and how and draw on some remarkable experiences of the work of palliative care professionals and hospices.

Sometimes, however, death comes unexpectedly, even suddenly – as with my own wife whilst I was writing my contributions to this book. In such cases, there is no time, or very little time, in which to talk about dying – so how do we handle that? How can we talk about 'sudden death'? This is the subject of chapter 5. In such cases, death may be the result of a car accident or an accident at work, at home, or during a holiday abroad. It may be the result of crime or war or a so-called 'natural disaster'. In these cases we are simply confronted with the stark reality of living without our loved one, our neighbour, our colleague. So how do we respond? And how do we deal with the difficult questions about who, if anyone, is to blame? Do we go into denial and try to carry on as if nothing has really changed? Or do we try to find someone who understands, with whom we can talk?

We next turn to two particular types of sudden death. In

chapter 6, we address the tragedy of suicide and how to cope with the practical and emotional issues it raises. And in chapter 7, we consider the death of a baby, either as a result of a miscarriage, stillbirth or, as in the case of my own son Andrew, during the very early hours or days of life.

With both suicide and the death of a baby, it is necessary to consider carefully how we talk about them to children as well as adults. In chapter 8, we also consider the particular challenges which come when a child is diagnosed with a terminal illness, and the additional emotional stresses which arise in that situation. How much should the child be told? When is the time to 'let go'? What about the different stages of childhood – from infancy to adolescence? What to say to other children – siblings, friends, classmates? And what to say to parents struggling with their own advance grief? Here we are privileged to draw on the expertise of the children's hospice movement and other agencies for dying and bereaved children, which have done so much to transform children's (and parents') experience of dying.

All the questions we have addressed so far raise the issue of what happens after death: is death 'the end' or is there life after it? In chapter 9, we consider the range of views, from the secular world and from the world of faith and, from the Christian perspective to what the Bible says about death, about heaven, and about hope.

Many people want to avoid talking or even thinking about death because they are afraid – afraid of pain, afraid of loss of control, afraid of the unknown, afraid of death itself. But this reluctance to engage has to be overcome when, as a result of an illness, a terminal diagnosis or the death of a loved one, the stark reality of dying and death confronts us. So in chapter 10 we consider how to face up to our fears, in their many dimensions. Here we draw on the experience of those in various counselling professions, as well as the significance of the Christian concept of hope.

We follow this in chapter 11 by considering how healing can come to our minds and spirits even as we face the dying of our bodies. In spite of the tremendous advances of medical science in recent decades, there remain limits to what medicine can achieve. This means that there comes a point when it has to be admitted that there is no prospect of 'cure' of our ailments. In that situation, the role of medicine, consultants, doctors, nurses and other carers changes. Its emphasis moves from 'cure' to 'care' – making the process of dying as comfortable and painless as possible.

At this point, particular difficulties may arise for people of faith. For example, what now is the role of prayer? How can we pray? For what can we pray? How can we bring hope to the dying and to loved ones? Will the absence of healing (in the sense of being cured) undermine faith?

In chapter 12 we turn to some of the practical questions which have to be tackled – putting your affairs in order, making preparations for an expected death, and what to do when someone dies at home. In addition to making a will, and the possible consequences of not doing so, there are questions of speaking to and/or seeing relatives and friends, and the need to 'make one's peace' with some. And, for many, this will be an opportunity to think about funeral arrangements.

In our final chapter, we return to the initial question of how we can help when someone is given the bleak news that they have a terminal illness. Here we offer some practical advice, and point to resources which can help, noting the variety of contexts in which these are needed – spouses, children, parents, other relatives, friends, colleagues, members of social groups like churches. How can we talk about it? What can we say and at what point? How do we say it? How do we deal with our emotions and struggles?

To accompany this, at the end of the book we provide an Appendix entitled '*More practical help*', containing further guidance as to where information can be found, followed by a Bibliography and list of additional websites.

Serious illness, dying and death itself pose profound questions, striking at the heart of what life is and our sense of identity. We do not pretend to provide all the answers in this book. But we do believe that, by encouraging *talking about dying*, we are offering a powerful way of helping one another as and when we have to face up to these questions and challenges. By showing that many have trodden these paths before us, by explaining and (we hope) de-mystifying the processes and procedures involved, by suggesting ways of making sensible preparation for what is bound to come, and by pointing to other resources which will be helpful to those in particular situations, we trust that this book will be both an encouragement and a source of hope to everyone, whatever their religious persuasion. We the authors are Christians who believe that experience confirms the truth of those ancient words of St Paul writing to the church in Rome: 'I am convinced that neither death nor life, neither angels nor demons, neither the present nor the future, nor any powers, neither height nor depth, nor anything else in all creation, will be able to separate us from the love of God that is in Christ Jesus our Lord' (Romans 8:38).

2

COPING WITH LIFE-THREATENING ILLNESS

Elaine Sugden

This chapter discusses the most difficult time when there is a new diagnosis of life-threatening illness. Cancer is the one that springs to most minds. Because I was a cancer doctor, many of my illustrations, but by no means all, are from cancer patients. There are other more unusual, life-threatening illnesses, some of which are so grave and rapid that there is no opportunity for the sort of reflection given here. The cause doesn't matter as the principles are the same. It is also important to remember that the term 'life-threatening' does not mean that untimely death is inevitable. Today, many are cured and treatment has given years of good quality survival to many others, but sadly not all.

The time of the diagnosis
The diagnosis of a disease which is life-threatening suddenly changes everything. Perhaps there had been fear that some recent symptoms might result in a serious diagnosis. For others, it comes out of the blue. There might not have been any symptoms, or the possibility of something serious had not been thought of. Having screening for diseases such as breast, prostate or bowel cancer is a worrying time for some, whilst for others it is just something routine. Most of those screened will not have the disease, but for the tiny minority who do, it is a devastating result.

Whatever has gone before the confirmation of the

diagnosis, the possibility of death sooner than expected is now centre stage in our thoughts. We leave the place where the news has been given in a daze, with questions unasked or unanswered. Much of what has been said was probably not heard. Nothing seems real, everything belongs to a dream world, which we long to wake from and find untrue.

The diagnosis of serious disease will not always lead to an early death, but at this stage the future is uncertain and has to be faced.

Why is death and dying such a problem even though it will happen to all of us? We shall certainly all die but few feel ready. Even the very elderly can find a life-threatening diagnosis hard to bear. Rightly and properly, there is a very strong human instinct to avoid death, to hang on to life, to put off death's inevitability and finality.

Fear is the major emotion in this situation. Fear about self, family, pain, the possibility of disability and of what might be beyond death. The uncertainty when treatment might or might not cure can be intolerable. Phases of denial, anger, guilt, and depression, in any order and for variable lengths of time can be experienced. Overwhelming feelings of disappointment and loss might occur as well as the unfairness of it all, prompting the cry 'why me?' There can be sleeplessness and dark dreams.

For some, the worst worry is about others rather than themselves.

Jill, a friend, soon after a cancer diagnosis, told me: 'As a person of faith I don't fear dying as such – although I am not very keen on pain – but I am terrified of leaving my husband. We have often talked about death in the abstract, and decided we would like to go together, as neither of us feels we would cope being the one left behind. I do really fear for how he would cope without me.'

Telling others

Not everyone has a trusted relative or friend with them when they are informed of the diagnosis, and some still prefer to keep it to themselves. Even husbands and wives do not always confide in each other, thinking that there will be time in the future to spill the beans. I would say, it is almost impossible to keep such important information from someone who cares about us without them realising that something is wrong. However hard it may seem, it is good to share information and talk about the diagnosis and its consequences. The truth can be easier to bear than the possibilities the imagination conjures up.

Jill again: 'My husband has surprised me with his willingness to face up to my diagnosis. He has never been one who copes well with illness, either his own or anyone else's. He has been hugely supportive so far, transporting me around to various hospitals and hanging around for hours waiting for me. I do feel proud of him – we have even discussed our Wills, which were drawn up many years ago and may need amending slightly. He wants to read all the literature I have been given.'

Telling others about the diagnosis is, for some, one of the most difficult things they will have to do. This is especially true in telling children who need to know that the disease is no one's fault, that it is not catching, that their questions will be answered honestly and, most of all, that they are loved and cared about. (This is explored further in chapter 8.)

Being ready to find that many, who want to help, are interested in our diagnosis is important.

'I said I was going to get cards printed up saying what kind of cancer I had and what treatment I needed. I know people cared, but I got sick and tired of repeating the same story every time someone asked...' Van, age 26

American Cancer Society – 'Telling others about your cancer'.[1]

Coming to terms with the diagnosis

'Coming to terms' with the diagnosis and the possibility of a shortened life span is made easier with kindness, care and support from others. The way in which we, and others, make use of the time we are given, is important.

Time: A healer

It is true that time is a great healer. In this sense, we are not talking about physical healing of the disease but coming to terms with the diagnosis and expectation of 'untimely' death. No one comes to terms with bad news within a few hours; it may take days, weeks or even months. But in the end most of us do.

Quote from a cancer survivor: 'There's a fear that goes through you when you are told you have cancer. It's so hard in the beginning to think about anything but your diagnosis. It's the first thing you think about every morning. Talking about your cancer helps you deal with all of the new emotions you are feeling. Remember, it's normal to get upset. I want people diagnosed with cancer to know it does get better.'

American Cancer Society:
'The emotional impact of a cancer diagnosis'.[2]

Time: For doctors, nurses and other health care staff to give explanations and support

Doctors, nurses and other health care staff need to dedicate adequate time towards carefully explaining the diagnosis, discovering the patient's priorities, showing care and offering continued support. This can help to calm fears about the illness and its treatment. Knowing the truth, and having confidence that the medical staff will be honest, is far more helpful than the false kindness of being shielded from a painful diagnosis.

In the situation where treatment will not be effective, time for full explanations and for the reassurance of continued physical and psychological care is especially important. Specialist nurses, who are trained to understand the particular disease and its psychological, as well as physical, effect on the patient are invaluable.

I think it is a good idea not to leave out your own GP. He or she is still your doctor. It was not unusual for my patients to admit to not seeing their own doctor because they were 'now under the hospital'. I encouraged them to visit their General Practitioner (GP) from time to time to keep in touch, and inform him/her about how things were going, as well as ensuring that medication for any symptoms or side effects were in place. Your doctor can encourage you, listen to your priorities for treatment and care, and help you to understand complex letters from the hospital which are full of medical jargon.

From a 32-year-old with a brain tumour who felt that the doctor had kept the full truth from him: 'People want truthful information and to be told what is expected to happen. The internet has been the best place for me to get information.'

'Living with Dying', healthtalk.org [3]

The internet is a useful source of information and we have suggested some websites at the end of this book. It is usually helpful to ask your doctor or specialist nurse about which sites they would recommend in light of your particular case. There is certainly no value in getting hold of wrong and possibly unnecessarily worrying information.

Time: From family, friends and communities

Receiving love and support from family members and friends is of the greatest value and importance. Most of us need company, and it can be devastating to be shunned by those who feel they don't know what to say. (No-one really knows what to say.) Just being present and available for whatever is needed is important, even if it is simply silent companionship. Other forms of love and support might include receiving invitations to outings, parties and other gatherings, or going to the pub, races, shopping, or a sports match together. It's good to be taken out of yourself. Often, practical help is also of great value. If you are the patient, do let others help – they really do want to. Tell them what would help you – it might be something they haven't thought of. If you are the relative or friend, be sure to ask how you can best help.

Faced with a difficult diagnosis, we want to feel that we still fit in with the family, our friends and interest groups. Whatever our situation, whenever possible, we want to continue to contribute our skills and pursue our interests and have a laugh. There are other things to talk about as well as illness.

Sometimes though, it does help to talk about the illness and the effect it is having. Whom you choose to speak to might surprise you.

> 'People share selectively with whichever individual or group they choose and might never 'open up' with their closest friends.'
>
> *When Your Friend is Dying*, Elizabeth Dean Burnham [4]

Time: For goals and interests

When the length of life is limited and a great deal of time is taken up with hospital visits it is helpful to think about what you would like to do with the time that is available. Having a purpose day by day is good therapy. Of course, energy might be limited and free time measured only in minutes, but it is worth planning for and trying to do something each day that you would expect to enjoy. This is, in fact, a good policy for all of us.

> A cancer patient attending a day hospice said: 'I have been involved in lots of different and interesting things, both in and outside the hospice, I wouldn't have been involved in if I hadn't had cancer.'
>
> 'Living with Dying', healthtalk.org [3]

Time: For renewing contact with family and friends

Often, there are people we have not seen for months or years that we desire to see and talk to. There will be some we want to thank for their love and friendship, maybe for something they did for us as a child, or as a young or older adult. Quite often, there have been family estrangements that need to be addressed. Forgiveness is a powerful force and the healing of broken relationships will provide comfort to all involved.

Dorothea had not seen or communicated with her daughter for 30 years. When in her mid-80s, she was ill and knew that death was not far off, she travelled alone across the Irish Sea to visit her daughter in England and say goodbye.

Ways of coping

'Coping' means: to face and deal with responsibilities, problems, or difficulties in a calm or adequate manner.

I worked as a cancer doctor for almost 30 years. It was clear that people coped with a difficult diagnosis in different ways, depending on their personality and background.

The active approach: 'I'm going to fight this, it's not going to get me.' Some people regain control in this way, determined to try to prove the doctors wrong. They intend to give it their best shot. However, sometimes a person might spend so much time looking for cures that they miss out on spending good and meaningful time with family and friends.

The passive approach: 'I'll do everything you tell me, doctor.' The feeling expressed here is that to follow medical advice 'to the letter' will bring the best result.

And the one I called 'head in the sand': 'I know I've got cancer and that one day I am going to die from it but I don't want to read books, leaflets or even talk about it; I want to enjoy life as long as I can.'

Those who took this approach often did not want to discuss the diagnosis even with the doctor and it could seem that they hadn't understood that their life was likely to be cut short.

Others look to a religious faith or alternative medicine to help them to cope.

> Mary held a strong belief in a God who cares. When her cancer returned, her doctor thought she didn't understand or was denying the situation. Mary was sure that she was in the hands of something more powerful than medicine.
>
> *The Art of Conversation through Serious Illness*,
> Richard P. McQuellon and Michael A Cowan [5]

'Coping' means regaining control of self and a continued purpose in life and this is an important step.

In my experience, no one way of coping is best or even better from the point of view of altering the course of the illness. Doctors, nurses, carers, family and friends must work with the sufferer and find out how best to help.

Having a purpose

For all of us the length of our lives is limited. There are things we want to do, places we want to go, and people we want to see during our life span. As life goes on, we change those 'wants' depending on money, time and priorities. After a difficult diagnosis, time is shorter and priorities can change; money might well be tighter but there are still opportunities. Rather than think about loss of hope, think instead about purpose and opportunity. Think through your dreams and hopes and make some choices – some may remain dreams, others will be less important than before, some will seem especially important and some, perhaps with the help of others, you will be able to achieve.

A patient was in her early 40s when a serious life-threatening illness was diagnosed. With treatment she lived just less than a year. In those months during her treatment she taught her husband and son to cook and look after themselves.

After her diagnosis Val was housebound. Her visitors invariably found that she gave them more encouragement and help than they gave her. She continued to have an important purpose in life.

A patient with motor neurone disease: 'I've got two choices. I can either spend my time worrying about the end or spend the time I have in living.'

'Living with Dying', healthtalk.org[3]

Some people have pointed out that after a life-threatening diagnosis they have appreciated nature, family, friends and all manner of things in a way they hadn't previously. This is the paradox of life enhancement when time might be limited.

A close friend told me: 'I signed a pre-operation form for a life-threatening operation accepting I might not wake up afterwards. Since waking up from it, every day has become a plus: what a privilege to be around to do this, that and the other.'

On the other hand, while some experience life enhancement others are 'paralysed' by uncertainty. Before a difficult diagnosis, uncertainty as to what might be wrong causes enormous anxiety. The relief at having an explanation for all the symptoms can then be replaced by the uncertainty for life itself 'Will the treatment work?' – 'How long have I got?' Some feel they could cope better if only they knew one way or the other. Such an accurate prediction is rarely possible. Uncertainty persists. This is part of 'coming to terms with' the reality of the diagnosis.

As time goes by

Many people talk about a roller coaster existence. Things seem to be going well, then there are setbacks: a worrying scan or other test, troublesome side effects from treatment or an unrelated other illness. These are all things to share with the medical team. It will help them, as well as you, to know your particular worries and hear your questions.

The most difficult time for some people is when a course of treatment comes to an end. During the course of treatment, they look forward to its completion and the freedom from any resulting side effects. However, when the hard slog of repeat treatments and side effects is over, they feel lonely and isolated. They miss the close involvement of the medical team.

Talking to someone who has been through this before can be very useful. Specialist nurses, patient support groups and agencies can also help. We have listed some of these at the end of this book. Talking about these anxieties will often help. Friends need to remember these normal but often unexpected emotions.

Continued fear

Sometimes I had patients who continued to suffer psychologically from uncertainly about the future even if treatment had gone well. Talking with the specialist nurse, the information centre, their doctor or counsellor helped some of them. Some needed prescribed medication to lift their mood.

A patient was in her 30s when she developed a rapidly growing rare tumour, wrapped around her neck, that was immediately life threatening and needed emergency chemotherapy. Although she responded to the treatment dramatically and fully, overwhelming anxiety that the tumour might come back made her unable to look after her 4-year-old child or her husband. Fortunately, but only after many months, she agreed to have antidepressants and as a result, after a few weeks, was able to start living again. The tumour did not come back.

Key Points

- A new life-threatening diagnosis is a common situation with common reactions
- Ways of coping vary and are equally valid
- There is great value in talking with the medical team, your GP and trusted family and friends
- If you are the person with the diagnosis try to remain positive, look for a daily purpose
- If you are family and friends, know that 'just being there' is helpful. No-one knows exactly what to say. Remember that even after the end of treatment support is needed and can be very helpful.

At the end of the book we have listed books and pamphlets you might find useful. There are also listed websites of information and support organisations that are regularly updated online.

Notes

[1] American Cancer Society: 'Telling others about your cancer' www.cancer.org/treatment/understandingyourdiagnosis/talkingaboutcancer/talking-with-friends-and-relatives-about-your-cancer (accessed May 2016).

[2] American Cancer Society: The emotional impact of a cancer diagnosis www.cancer.org/treatment/treatmentsandsideeffects/emotionalsideeffects/copingwithcancerineverydaylife/a-message-of-hope-emotional-impact-of-cancer (accessed May 2016).

[3] 'Living with Dying' (healthtalk.org) recorded interviews with people with life-threatening illnesses, introduced by Dawn French: www.healthtalk.org/peoples-experiences/dying-bereavement/living-dying/topics (accessed May 2016).

[4] Burnham, Elizabeth Dean, *When your Friend is Dying* (Kingsway Publications, 1983) Chapter 3.

[5] McQuellon, Richard P, and Cowan, Michael A, *The Art of Conversation through Serious Illness* (Oxford University Press, 2010) p19.

3

DIFFICULT DECISIONS

Elaine Sugden

Most of us are apprehensive when seeing a hospital doctor, particularly if we have never met the doctor before. It is good to take a relative or friend with you into the appointment. This person can help you remember things you wanted to ask, and make a note of important things you are told.

Try to arrive in good time; parking and finding your way around a hospital can take longer than you think. Take a list of any questions you have and ask for anything you do not understand to be repeated and explained. Hospitals are aware of patients' needs and provide a Patient Advice and Liaison Service (PALS for short), which can help if you have ongoing concerns about the medical process.

Deciding about treatment

Decisions by doctors about a person's treatment will, whenever possible, be a joint decision with that person (together with family or friends, if the person wishes). The opportunity to accept or decline medical treatment will normally be given both at initial diagnosis and when treatment is no longer helpful. The patient and their families will usually be given appropriate information and sensitive help when deciding which option to choose.

Most of us with a serious illness will want to have treatment. But before making a decision, it is important to find out how effective the treatment is likely to be, whether it will cure or not and what the side effects would be. Sometimes, for example, in the very elderly, the treatment itself can be too severe to be given safely and this reduces the options available to the patient.

Sometimes there are choices to be made between one treatment and another. Increasingly, doctors are asking patients to decide between different treatments, or to choose between opting for treatment or not. This can be overwhelmingly difficult for some patients who would prefer a doctor they can trust to make the decision for them. When one treatment is likely to be as useful as another, there might be one that is more suited to you and your lifestyle. It is difficult to make an on-the-spot decision. Usually, there is time to take the information sheets away and have a discussion with any family and friends you wish. It is important to consult your GP, who will have the experience and wisdom to help you. Remember though that the final decision is yours and you must feel content about it.

When there is no longer any useful treatment/ stopping treatment

Sadly, a time may come when there are no further treatment options for the doctor to suggest. Doctors have been trained to put things right. Death at the end of treatment is not the outcome they want and they may feel they have failed. They may assume patients would rather not discuss death. There is a fear, even among doctors, that talking about it will hasten death or make someone lose hope. In fact, neither of these fears is true and patients are often helped by the honesty of truthful information. Many doctors are not good at talking about death. Too often they do not tell patients and their families when death is approaching. It is a subject that we all find difficult, but need to discuss. It is good to talk.

Peter, a member of my family, was 54 when he was found to have severe spinal arthritis reducing the movement and feeling of his legs. An operation was advised, which turned into several operations because the wounds would not heal. He was in intensive care. His legs would not work at all. His memory was affected so that, although he could have a conversation, it was forgotten within seconds. In spite of family intervention and against their wishes, his doctor insisted on continuing with operations and medication and in the end Peter died while still being investigated.

It makes sense, therefore, for doctors and other medical staff to find out what patients and their families actually want in the last days/weeks/months of life, when treatment has virtually no chance of bringing about any improvement. A discussion gives the opportunity for active treatment to be stopped, and for proper palliative care to be provided. Palliative care aims to manage symptoms such as pain and make the process of dying as comfortable as possible and any attempts to change the progress of the disease are stopped. This means that patients who do not wish to pursue active treatment can do what is important to them rather than having to visit the hospital repeatedly and deal with side effects of treatment. (See chapter 4 for more about palliative care.)

A GP wrote to me: 'It is not unusual for patients to come to see me asking (or seeking permission) to decline further intervention, especially chemotherapy. Patients can feel pressured into treatment because the doctor feels that it would be a failure not to be able to treat further, or treatment is bound to be what the patient wants, or that they will be criticised if they don't, or for research interests. Sometimes treatment is not in the patient's best interests and actually can get in the way of accepting and planning death.'

Is treatment ever denied or stopped because of expense?
Treatments that have been shown to have definite benefit are almost always available for use. But some treatments are extremely expensive, and I have often heard patients and families ask if they are being denied treatment because of cost. In my experience, the usual reason for refusing to give a particular treatment is that it has not been fully tested to ensure that it is sufficiently safe for use. In the UK, we are very privileged to have the National Health Service (NHS) as well as world-class medical research. The National Institute of Clinical Excellence (NICE)[1] is the part of the NHS that is responsible for setting out compulsory standards for medical services, so that they are not only safe but of the highest quality, as well as being cost effective. If the benefit of a treatment is likely to be very slight, it might be thought not worth either its financial or toxicity (severe side effects) costs. Many treatments compete for the limited resources of the NHS: vaccines for children, care for older people, accident and emergency for the whole population, as well as treatment for cancer and many chronic diseases. All must be provided for. Sometimes difficult decisions do have to be made.

Cardio Pulmonary Resuscitation (CPR) [2]

Sometimes the heart stops suddenly, for instance, after a heart attack or drowning. It must be started up within very few minutes to avoid death. In this situation, there is no time for discussion or choice. Action must be immediate.

Doctors in the 1950s developed a way of trying to restart the heart (i.e. resuscitate someone) after a sudden 'death'. Since the 1970s, the general public has been encouraged to learn this way of controlling the breathing and keeping the heart pumping until there is medical help.

This is always worth trying but is not always successful; nor is it without risk. In hospital, even where immediate medical help is available, resuscitation is often not successful and afterwards less than one in ten leave hospital. Those with advanced life-threatening disease (e.g. cancer) are extremely unlikely to be satisfactorily resuscitated. Similarly, information on the very elderly indicates that only one in every twenty people resuscitated in nursing homes and then transferred to hospital ever leave hospital again. Some who do start breathing again never regain consciousness or cannot live without medical machines, and some are brain damaged.

Do Not Attempt Resuscitation (DNAR) Directive/Decision

In the course of a patient's treatment, many medical choices and decisions have to be made. In some cases, doctors may conclude that the patient's serious condition is not responding and will not respond to further treatment. In that event, although death may not be imminent, doctors might suggest that, when the heart and breathing do stop, resuscitation as described above should not be attempted. The patient should be allowed to die naturally. This is something for doctors and their patients and families to decide together.

A GP or a hospital doctor can ask the patient, or the patient can ask the doctor about this. Together, they decide whether a Do Not Attempt Resuscitation (DNAR) directive is reasonable. Without this directive, an ambulance is called and full attempted resuscitation is started. This involves repeated pressure on the chest, fluid drips, artificial breathing and electrical stimulation to the body. If it does not work this is not a nice way to die. For most of us it would be better to die in peace.

> Two weeks ago, as I write this, a close family member aged 90 collapsed in her nursing home where she was becoming increasingly frail. She had been reluctant to sign that she did not want resuscitation and so full resuscitation was started and continued in the ambulance. She did not survive the journey. She did not have the peaceful death I had wished for her.

Similarly, in hospital, however ill or elderly the patient, resuscitation procedures will be carried out unless they and their doctor have previously agreed that this should not be done.

Advanced Decision/Directive (see also Appendix 3)
Equally difficult, but very helpful, is to have what is called an Advanced Directive or Advanced Decision, also known as a 'Living Will'. This is a signed document which lists what you would *not* want to happen to you in the event of an immediately life-threatening event. It is something you can do to influence a medical decision in the future. It enables you to think about what you would like to happen if you lose the ability to take informed decisions about your care. Examples of such decisions include: artificial feeding, cardio pulmonary resuscitation and life-saving treatment

when the brain has been damaged, after a stroke, head injury or dementia.

Considering an advanced directive also provides an opportunity for you to decide if you would or would not want to donate your organs.[3]

Often, people have seen family or friends kept alive by doctors, rather than being 'allowed to die' naturally, and many people do not like to think they might die whilst connected to life-sustaining tubes and other equipment.

E. was a very special and loved wife, mother, aunt, great aunt and grandmother. In her 80s she had a stroke and initially was not expected to survive. Although she was unable to communicate in any way, the doctors gave her a permanent feeding tube that kept her alive in a nursing home for many months. She was unable to speak or give any indication that she understood what was being said. Her family were sure she would not have wanted to be in this condition at the end of life.

It is important to tell your family about any of these decisions that you make so that, if you are suddenly in this situation, they can tell medical staff. If the doctors involved do not know about this decision, they will attempt resuscitation and other measures to continue life.

Power of Attorney

If you are reaching the time when you might need help with decision-making, then you should think about who you want to appoint to do this for you. This is called a Power of Attorney and is explained in chapter 12: *Practical Matters*.

Decisions for the elderly

Improvements in social and economic conditions, and particularly in medical science, have resulted in more of us living until we are over 80 and many well beyond that.

None of us is going to last forever, but the timing of death depends on our genes, lifestyle, gender, and many other personal factors, both known and unknown. Although we hear about remarkable 90 or 100 year-olds, most people at these advanced ages are not able to live independently and many need a great deal of care. The inevitability of decline for those of us fortunate enough to live into very old age has been said to be the price we pay for living longer.

A doctor in an affluent part of America spoke about some of his patients: 'They think they'll always be able to play strenuous sports or travel anywhere they want to or continue working twelve hours a day. They assume if something goes wrong I'll be able to fix it. But one day they're going to wake up and discover they can't do everything they once did. Someday they'll be old and they won't like it because they're not emotionally prepared for it.'[4]

So we need to be realistic about the future. Whatever age you are and health you are in as you read this, now is the time to make sure you have an up-to-date Will. Distribution of your money, property and possessions needs to be thought about in time. The majority of us in the UK have not made a Will although more than half of over-55-year-olds have done so. (See chapter 12: *Practical Matters*.)

'But I still have not signed my Will, because it is thought provoking and sad. Seeing my Last Will and Testament, bound in card and bearing my name, was a strange, almost out-of-body, experience. But equally, as soon as it is signed I can put it in a drawer and concentrate on living. Maybe it is not such a big deal after all.'[5]

Make your choices before it is too late and make sure your family know your wishes so that, in the event of a life-threatening emergency, they can tell the medical staff. If doctors don't know your wishes, they will definitely start resuscitation efforts.

In this chapter, I have tried to provide straightforward information to help those with a serious illness and their relatives in coping with what may seem daunting experiences. To conclude, I have set out the key points:

Key Points from this chapter

- It is usual today for doctors, nurses and others in health care to encourage patients to take part in making decisions about their own health and care. This is particularly necessary in the areas described in this chapter.
- Having someone you trust with you when seeing a doctor for important decisions is recommended.
- When cure has not occurred and treatment against the disease is no longer helping, a change to palliative care might provide more benefit.
- Resuscitation is unlikely to be successful in those who are frail from illness or advanced years. In these cases, a Do Not Attempt Resuscitation directive is appropriate.
- We will all die. However, none of us knows when sudden completely unexpected death might occur. Less than one in ten deaths are sudden and without warning.
- Even if you are fit and well the preparation of an Advanced Decision or Directive is encouraged. (See Appendix 3.)
- A Power of Attorney gives a person of your choosing the responsibility for your medical decisions and financial affairs, when you are unable. It can be drawn up now

and brought into effect when needed – see chapter 12: *Practical Matters*.

- Making a Will is something we can do that will help those left behind – see chapter 12: *Practical Matters*.

Notes

[1] National Institute for Health and Care Excellence (NICE): www.nice.org.uk/

[2] Resuscitation Council (UK): www.resus.org.uk/

[3] NHS organ donation web site:

www.organdonation.nhs.uk/register-to-donate/

for medical purposes in the event of your death

[4] Graham, Billy, *Nearing Home, Life, Faith and Finishing Well* (Thomas Nelson, 2011), pp7-8.

[5] Lucy Townsend, *BBC News Magazine*, 19 October, 2011.

Other resources

Gawande, Atul, *Being Mortal* (Profile Books, Wellcome Collection, 2014).

Mack, Jennifer W. and Smith, Thomas J., 'Reasons why clinicians do not have discussions about poor prognosis, why it matters and what can be improved', American Cancer Society, 2012

http://jco.ascopubs.org/content/30/22/2715.full.pdf+html

Worth, Jennifer, *In the Midst of Life* (Weidenfeld & Nicolson, 2012).

4

TALKING ABOUT DYING:
WHEN, WHERE AND HOW?

Elaine Sugden

Growing old

Whilst 70 ('three score years and ten') used to be the expected life span, with modern medicine this is now not so. We are living longer and, at the time of writing, the commonest age at death for men is 85 and for women 89 whilst many live into their hundreds.[1] Most of us agree that living into these later years is fine if we are fit and well, but that is the exception not the rule and few very elderly people are independent. Of course, it helps to keep active and eat sensibly but even so, as the years go by, our bodies wear out and do not repair as they did when we were younger. Ageing begins from the moment of birth. Few of us choose exactly when we die but, without exception, for everyone who is born the time to die will come. Although there is a right and proper human instinct for survival, we cannot beat death forever.

Around 500,000 people die in England each year. Today in the UK, death in old age is the rule rather than the exception. With an increasingly ageing population, the majority of older people will be living with a number of medical conditions and 1 in 6 of those over 80 have dementia.[2] The art is to live well until the end.

> 'For those living into the years of frailty, it is important to have goals and a purpose, to know what you are fighting for.'[3]

The limits of modern medicine

We live in the hope that modern medicine will always put us right. When I was training in medical school in the 1970s, heart attacks were a common cause of death. Now, because of a reduction in smoking, as well as the availability of medicines to reduce the risk and operations to improve the heart's blood supply, sudden death from heart attack is much less common. Cancer is still known to be a great killer, but medical progress has improved cure rates and increased the length of remissions so that we expect, even after a diagnosis of incurable cancer, to have several years of life before death. Whilst we feel well, we can't imagine any of these things happening to us.

'At bottom no one believes in his own death, which amounts to saying: In the unconscious each of us is convinced of his own immortality'

Sigmund Freud, in *Reflections on War and Death* [4]

Some very elderly people who are medically rescued from death never regain independence, or are never able to communicate with others or enjoy life in any way again. In cases like this, the only purpose in living is to keep the enemy (death) at bay.

Artificial feeding can maintain this difficult situation for months or even a year or more. Perhaps it is such people that physician-assisted suicide is thought to help? But wouldn't it have been better not to prolong life artificially in the first place?

Most of us dread this happening to us. The only way we can try to prevent it is to complete an Advanced Directive (see chapter 3: *Difficult Decisions* and Appendix 3) and tell our family/friends about our wishes.

'Death is not of course a failure, death is normal – medicine fails the people it is trying to help (by its) intrusive treatments. (We are) victims of our refusal to accept the inevitability of decline and death.'

Atul Gawande, *Being Mortal*[5]

'Medical intervention can keep someone alive in such a state that it is very difficult to answer the question whether they are dying or not. Sometimes it is the family who are holding out for a cure and encouraging the patient to continue with any treatment offered.'

Atul Gawande, *Being Mortal*[6]

Lack of care can be even worse.

A much-loved uncle of mine lived until he was 99. Towards the very end of his life, he had been in and out of hospital and patched up several times. The time he died he had not been looked after as well as usual. He had been moved between hospitals, left alone and uncared for, his family not knowing where he was. It was many years before his daughter could think about the times he had been well looked after in hospital because of the picture in her mind of his dying state.

Cicely Saunders, founder of the hospice movement, wrote: 'How we die remains in the memory of those who live on.'

Fears about dying

The most often quoted fear about dying is that it will be painful, or at least that the time leading up to death will be painful. Some fear dying in hospital. Some fear dying alone. Many fear mostly for family and friends, and worry about how they will cope, especially if there is a dependent relative or friend. Most say they don't mind dying, but don't want pain or other problems that might come before death. Only a few admit to being anxious about what might, if anything, happen after death. (Chapter 9: *Talking about Life after Death* explores this further.) Over half the deaths in the UK are in hospital; families often keep a long vigil at the bedside, anxious that their relative should not die alone.

Palliative/hospice-type care of the dying

It must be true to say that we all hope to die without pain. Physical pain can almost always be controlled with the modern use of morphine-type pain medicines that leave the person fully conscious and alert. It is important for all doctors and nurses to learn the skill of using these medicines.

The hospice movement, pioneered by Dame Cicely Saunders who founded St Christopher's Hospice in London UK, one of the first hospices, made control of pain and other symptoms a founding principle. 'Palliative care' has become a well-known phrase and describes treatment, not against the disease itself, but to control the symptoms produced by the disease. 'Active treatment' (aimed at controlling the disease) and palliative treatments (to reduce symptoms such as pain, breathlessness, nausea) need to be used together, until active treatment is no longer able to help or make a difference. Then, palliative treatment, often called 'palliative care' can take over fully.

To some people, replacing treatment aimed at cure or prolonging life with palliative care means that the doctors are giving up on their treatment and even abandoning them. It can be hard to leave the care of a doctor who has worked hard over the years to keep you well, and has become a trusted friend. In fact, further active treatment could do more harm than good, and the palliative care team is likely to make a worthwhile difference to quality of life. It is not unusual for a patient to live longer than expected once 'holistic' (all-round) care is underway.

'Patients worry about stopping treatment even if new symptoms are occurring and treatment is obviously not working. Doctors worry about denying treatment that just might give the patient more life. And so it continues and the confrontation with the much more likely death probability is deferred. We imagine that we can wait until the doctors tell us there is nothing more they can do, but doctors can almost always do something. When should they stop?'

Cancer Care study, *JAMA* (an international medical journal)

'Pushing on with more treatment when the chance of response is very low and the risk of troublesome side effects is high can remove the opportunity to prepare for the death that is inevitable. In general doctors overestimate a patient's survival time, they don't like to be unduly pessimistic and talking about death is difficult.'

Atul Gawande, *Being Mortal*[7]

If you could choose – How would you like to die?

Richard Smith, a doctor and former *British Medical Journal* editor, suggested four ways.[8]

- A sudden death – which many of us would choose for ourselves. But most people who have experienced this in a close relative or friend know that it is very difficult for those left behind, with no time to say all the things they think they would have said, including 'goodbye'.
- The long slow death of dementia – definitely not favoured by those who have experienced it in family or friend.
- The 'up and down' death of organ failure, often in hospital or seeing doctors.
- A cancer death where you are often reasonably in control for a shorter or longer time to do some of the things you wish to do before, what is often, a fairly speedy end.

Dr Smith said in his article that he preferred a cancer death. There were a lot of responses to his article. The fact is, we do not choose.

'My husband died 6 months ago from a sudden massive heart attack while cycling. I did not get to say goodbye, tell him I loved him one more time or hold his hand one more time. I have recently befriended a woman whose husband likely has little time left. We do not wish our fates on each other, nor do we compete on who is suffering the most. That is not the point but we do need to have these conversations'.

The response of one reader of Richard Smith's article:
'Dying of Cancer is the Best Death'

Dementia

Those who have witnessed dementia in a close relative or friend fear this decline more than any other. Those developing dementia of any sort usually realise only too well what is happening to them. Fortunately, today there is more general awareness of this condition, which is important to acknowledge and seek help for at an early stage. In some cases, medication can have an effect on the progress of the disease. Even so, conversations need to be had, so that the sufferer can decide whom he/she would like to make decisions, on their behalf, when they can no longer do that for themselves. A Lasting Power of Attorney (LPA) can give someone you trust the legal authority to make decisions on your behalf. This can then be implemented at a later stage if you lack mental capacity or no longer wish to make decisions for yourself. (See chapter 12, *Practical Matters*.)

For a person of ripe years to die in sleep or in a chair couldn't be bettered. My mother did just that but only after 30 years of progressive Alzheimer's dementia – not inaptly called a 'living death' – of self if not body.

A different sort of pain

For most people nearing death, pain can be controlled. The knowledge of how to use medicines against pain has been pioneered by the hospice movement and has spread throughout the UK, and the rest of the world. However, there is still a long way to go before every doctor and nurse understands the use of these medicines. More difficult to control is the 'psychological pain' that doesn't respond to medicines or other ways of controlling physical symptoms.

Psychological, mental or emotional pain can be severe and uncontrollable. This type of pain needs a different approach because it comes from anxiety about unhealed loss, guilt, scarred relationships or other deep hurts. Spiritual concerns, which can be closely related to emotional concerns, are also able to produce very real pain. (See chapter 9: *Talking about Life after Death* and chapter 10: *Facing up to Fear*). Hospices provide holistic (all-round) care to meet the physical, social, psychological and spiritual needs of patients and those of their family and friends.

'Sometimes the right medicine isn't medicine at all – and the most important skill is in knowing how to talk to someone.'[9]

Access to hospice care

There are hospices in or near most towns and cities throughout the country. But sadly, it is not possible for all who want to do so to die in a hospice. Hospices have more generous staffing numbers than hospitals and so are expensive to run. In general, most of their funding comes from charitable giving. In this way, whilst they must still have government Quality Reviews,[10] they are independent of the National Health Service and can run as they wish.

The 2013 figures suggest that only 7% of us say we want to die in hospital whereas half of us in fact do.[11]

Many of the patients I treated for cancer wanted to die in the hospice. For some this was possible, but for others, it was not possible because when they reached the last few weeks of life, the hospice beds were full. What can be offered is good palliative care at home (where 67% say they want to die) or in hospital (where half do die) and efforts are being made to make sure this is possible, usually through Macmillan or other community nurses. Hospice-type care is brought into the home, nursing home or hospital.

It is easier for cancer patients to access palliative care than for those with other diseases. It is important that good palliative care/end-of-life care becomes available for all.

Dying at home

Given the choice, a lot of people would prefer to die in their own home, surrounded by those they love. And some cases of sudden death take place in the home. When death does occur at home, it is important to know just what to do. A checklist for this is provided in Appendix 1: *Preparing for an expected death at home*.

The 'Dying matters' website[12] asks four questions to help you think:

- *Where do you want to die?* – at home, in a hospice, in a hospital, in a care home, or somewhere else?
- *When you are approaching the end of your life, is there anything you want to do?* – do you have a list of these, a 'bucket list'?
- *When you are approaching the end of your life, how do you want to be cared for?* – What medical support do you want? Are there any medical procedures or treatments you don't want? Do you have a preference for who cares for you? Do you want any spiritual support (i.e. support related to meaning and purpose, whether you are religious or non-religious)?
- *What do you want to happen after you have died?* What sort of funeral do you want? Do you want your organs to be donated to help others to live? Do you want to donate your body to science? Have you made a Will, is it up to date and where is it?

Physician assisted suicide

Those wanting euthanasia or physician-assisted suicide for themselves do not fear death, but want to control it or control their experience of, or fear of, unbearable symptoms or dependency on others. We have become used to having choice in most areas of life. Should we also have a choice in how and when we die? Fears of pain and dependency, as well as the exercise of choice at the end of life, are driving the increased pressure for euthanasia and doctor-assisted suicide.

These are the meanings of the terms regularly used when discussing this topic:

- **Euthanasia:** is the intentional killing by act or omission of a person whose life is thought not to be worth living.
- **Physician/Doctor assisted suicide:** is intentional medical killing where the final act is performed by the patient.
- **The withdrawal of treatment** that is futile or burdensome, or where the person is actively dying, is good medical care and should not be confused with euthanasia.
- **The use of strong pain medication at the end of life**, given to relieve symptoms, might hasten death but is not given for that reason and is not euthanasia.

The legal situation

Different countries have different legal rules. At the time of writing, most countries, in common with the UK, have not changed their law; euthanasia and physician-assisted suicide are still prohibited. Although some doctors in the UK are in favour of being able to assist patients to end their lives when death is expected within six months, at present the majority are not. Doctors and health workers, trusted as healers, do not wish this change in their role. However, in some countries, physician assisted suicide by lethal injection is now legal. In Belgium there has been gradual widening of eligibility for this ending of life; children of any age, with parental consent, are now included.

Circumstances can leave a person alive but without full consciousness or the ability to interact, with only artificial feeding and/or breathing sustaining life. Withdrawal of this life-sustaining technology usually has to be tested in the courts before it can be carried out legally.

'Compassion and dignity'

Those who wish for the legalisation of assisted suicide stress 'compassion' and 'dignity'. But concerns remain. What will be the pressure on the lonely elderly, recently bereaved or depressed to seek death? What about those who lack the capacity required for consent?

Compassion and dignity are indeed essential components of dying well and are needed all along the way, from a difficult diagnosis through tough treatment and into the terminal phase. Compassion from family and carers, and dignity in the way they are treated, are also needed in the care of the elderly as they reach their final years.

Interviewer to David Attenborough in the context of discussion of assisted suicide:[13]

'Do you think people should have the right to take their own life?'

'Yes, I suppose I do as long as you can solve all the problems associated with misuse of that right.'

As good a death as possible

Depending on our beliefs, backgrounds and personalities we look on the issues differently. There is, however, general agreement that each individual death should be made as good as it can be, remembering that each person is part of a wider family and community. Dying and death are never easy for the dying person or those close to them, accompanied as they can be, by pain and anxiety on part of both the dying person and their family, lack of or insufficient medication or sudden death leaving so much unsaid and no goodbyes. There is no 'perfect' death, not least because there are those left who deeply grieve and those who were out of reach at the time but who wanted to have said their last goodbyes.

How can we make dying as good as it can be in each situation? Those of us who believe that life is given by the God who commanded: 'you shall not kill' (Exodus 20:13), regard euthanasia or assisted suicide as wrong and unacceptable. Arguments in favour of legalising both procedures focus largely on the need to show 'compassion' by addressing the suffering of dying patients. Proponents argue that it is kinder to allow patients to end their lives prematurely than to force them to live with unbearable pain. However, distressing symptoms (such as severe pain) can be effectively managed through the provision of high-quality palliative care, making assisted suicide and euthanasia unnecessary. The Royal College of Psychiatrists has agreed that with proper palliative care, it is possible for patients to 'die with dignity'.[14]

Rather than licensing doctors to dispense lethal drugs, the most compassionate response to suffering would be to improve standards of palliative care and make it available to all those who need it. Such care also gives an opportunity for love and care to be shown to a loved one who is dying.

'My wife was told by our family doctor that I would die a painful death within 3 months. I wished for euthanasia – my death is inevitable – (but) since coming under the care of the Macmillan Service my pain has been relieved, my ability to enjoy life restored and my fears of an agonising end allayed. I am still alive today – I am living a full life.'[15]

> ·The aim is a good life to the end – assisted living is harder than assisted death.'
>
> Atul Gawande, *Being Mortal*[16]

> 'You matter because you are you. You matter to the last moment of your life and we will do all we can, not only to help you die peacefully but to live until you die.'
>
> Cicely Saunders, founder of the hospice movement

Purposeful Living

> 'For those of us coming nearer to the end of life, our steps may well be slow but they need not be without purpose.'
>
> Billy Graham, *Nearing Home: Life, Faith and Finishing Well*[17]

In the years when health, and particularly energy, is declining there are still things to be done to give a purpose to life. Spending time with grandchildren or other young people is of great value both to you and to them. Tell your stories and, if possible, write them down before it is too late. Meet with others for meals, to watch the television, listen to the radio or play games. Face-to-face communication has been shown to improve well-being and keep the mind active much more than the TV or a computer screen - and this goes for children as well as adults.

> 'In those last weeks or days people share memories, pass on wisdom and keepsakes, settle relationships, establish their legacies, make peace with God and ensure that those left behind will be OK. This is important both for the dying and those left behind.'   Atul Gawande[18]

Many families have unhealed relationships. Now that you are reading, thinking and perhaps talking about death, this is the time to do everything you can to bring healing to those relationships. Forgiveness is not easy but it is very powerful. You and others involved do not want to live with regrets.

How do we die?

When asked how we would like to die, most of us say that we would like to die suddenly. Not all agree and some would like time for goodbyes and making arrangements. Up-to-date records in the UK show that, of all people who die, less than one death in ten is sudden. Most deaths (more than nine out of every ten) occur after a variable period of illness, with gradual deterioration before a dying phase at the end. During these last hours the person seems to withdraw from life, their breathing becomes shallow, their voice weak and although the breathing may sometimes become noisy, in general they just fade away.

In her book *In the Midst of Life*, Jennifer Worth – also author of *Call the Midwife* – on several occasions speaks about the time of death:

> 'To be present at the time of death can be one of the most important moments of life. To see those last awesome moments of transition from life into death can only be described as a spiritual experience. And then afterwards, when the body lies still, one gets the strange feeling that the person has simply gone away, as though he/she has said "I'm just going into the other room. I'll leave that thing there while I'm gone, I won't be needing it".'[19]

It is not possible to predict accurately when death will occur. Some patients may appear to wait for someone to visit or for an important event, such as a birthday or a special holiday, and then die soon afterward. Others experience unexplained improvements and live longer than expected. A few seem to decide to die and do so very quickly, sometimes within minutes.

Care provided during those last hours and days can have profound effects, not just on the patient but on all present, including both family and professional caregivers at the very end of life. There is no second chance to get it right.

Key points from this chapter
- Life expectancy is increasing.
- Modern medicine has helped to postpone death in the elderly so that more are living with increasing frailty and dependency. It is important to have thought about and made some preparation for death.
- In general, natural death can be: sudden, a result of organ failure, because of cancer or with dementia – but we do not choose.
- Death and dying are not easy. There is no perfect death but each death should be made as good as possible.
- Palliative care can be used alongside active treatment and can improve quality of life by the control of pain and other symptoms. Used well, it can ensure as good a death as possible and allow the patient to die with dignity.
- The withdrawal of treatment that is no longer useful or is causing distress, or the use of strong medicines to control pain at the end of life are not active euthanasia.
- It is important to have a purpose for living even in the years of frailty.
- Care at the end of life and how we die is extremely important. There is no second chance to get it right.

Notes

[1] Office of National Statistics (ONS) http://ons.gov.uk/

[2] Dying Matters website www.dyingmatters.org/
Alzheimer's Society statistics: www.alzheimers.org.uk/statistics.

[3] Andrew Marr, Radio 4, Start the Week, 10.11.14, A Good Death.

[4] Sigmund Freud, in: *Reflections on War and Death*, translated by A A Brill and Alfred B Kuttner (New York: Moffat, Yard and Co., 1918).

[5] Gawande, Atul, *Being Mortal*, (London: Profile Books, 2014), pp8-10

[6] Ibid., p156.

[7] Gawamde, Atul, op. cit., p 167

[8] Richard Smith BMJ online blog: http://blogs.bmj.com/bmj/2014/12/31/richard-smith-dying-of-cancer-is-the-best-death/

[9] Napp (pharmaceutical company) advertisement in *British Medical Journal*, 13th April 2013.

[10] Care Quality Commission: www.cqc.org.uk

[11] Public Health England. What we know now 2013. New information collated by the National End of Life Care Intelligence Network.

[12] www.dyingmatters.org

[13] Radio 4, Costing the Earth, 18th November, 2015

[14] 'RCP cannot support legal change on assisted dying – survey results' http://bit.ly/1qj04Xf

[15] Cancer patient writing to World in Action Team 1980 – 8 months after diagnosis (in *A Time to Die*, Robert Twycross, Christian Medical Fellowship, 1994.)

[16] Gawande, Atul, op. cit., p2

[17] Graham, Billy, *Nearing Home: Life, Faith and Finishing Well* (Thomas Nelson, 2011), p130

[18] Gawande, Atul, op. cit., p249

[19] Worth, Jennifer, *In the Midst of Life* (London: Weidenfeld & Nicholson, 2010).

Other resources

Planning for your future care NHS Improving Quality (online only) discuses Advanced Care Planning and Advanced Directives:
www.ncpc.org.uk/sites/default/files/planning_for_your_future_updated_sept_2014%20%281%29.pdf

5

COPING WITH THE UNEXPECTED

Philip Giddings

No warning

'If only we had had time to talk.' Death does not always give warning. One of the most moving aspects of 9/11 was the recording of airline passengers speaking their final words to their loved ones as the planes hurtled towards their targets. If only we had had more time. For the victims of the London bombings in 2005, as movingly shown in the television programme *A Song for Jenny*,[1] there was no time to talk at all: the relatives and friends of many had to wait for days hoping against hope that the worst had not happened. The deaths were all the more agonising because they were arbitrary as well as horrific. There was no time to prepare.

What to say?

Apparent arbitrariness is also a feature of the deaths in traffic accidents or accidents at places of work, and these can be horrific too. What can we say to those experiencing the agony of such a bereavement? Words seem necessary, yet inadequate. Many of us find that we are struggling ourselves to articulate our feelings. These are circumstances in which simple presence with the bereaved and, when appropriate, the touch or an arm around the shoulder say more, and more adequately, than anything that words can convey. This was certainly my own experience when my wife died suddenly in October 2015.

A climbing accident

Part of the agony in such cases is the suddenness with which our world is turned upside down by the news of the loved one's death. Derek and Mary[2] were about to help with the catering for an Alpha group in their church when a phone call came through with news of a horrible accident. Their eldest son Michael was training to be a doctor. He and a group of his friends decided to take a few days break climbing in Spain. He loved climbing. But during the climb a rope broke loose and Michael fell to his death. A popular and gifted young man snatched away.

The effects on family

Derek and Mary were in different places when the first phone message came. They did not know whether each other knew. And they had to tell Michael's brothers and sisters, one doing his A-levels. They were understandably distraught. As Michael was living away from home doing his hospital training, there was the added complication of telling his friends. Derek felt numb. Mary initially could not take it in, experiencing a kaleidoscope of emotions, jagged bits and pieces of memory. She felt as if her brain was shutting down.

The intrusions

For Derek and Mary, numb as they both felt, life had to go on. They had, in particular, to care for their other children. They had to cope with visitors and the likelihood of press interest – one reporter 'just turned up on their doorstep'. These were the early days of Facebook so the news and reactions to Michael's sudden and tragic death spread rapidly in that medium – but for Derek and Mary this was their first encounter with social media. Feeling emotionally numb, Mary could not face driving: she did not feel safe. In fact, she did not like going out at daytime or shopping in the supermarket as she did not want to meet people.

The practicalities

Getting to grips with the practical things that had to be done was 'a killer'. Michael had no life insurance and, as the climbing trip was a 'spur of the moment' idea, he had no travel insurance either. Anxieties about arrangements for his body to be brought back to England were relieved when the undertakers took care of what needed to be done. As Michael had no longer been living at home, in addition to the funeral, there was a thanksgiving service to be organised in the town where he was training. They received so many cards that the postman enquired, embarrassingly, why they had so much post all of a sudden. They read the cards a few at a time. They were also sent lots of cuttings about Michael: Mary found this difficult and put them in a big box – and they were still there several years later.

'Goodbye' events

Mary and Derek were very grateful for the support they received from their local church, and from their vicar in particular. He visited them several times, did not stay long, and 'made no attempt to gush'. Having a son of a similar age, he had some understanding of what they were going through. Discussing the funeral was a challenge. Mary did not want the coffin to be in church, so there was a service at the crematorium for family and close friends, followed by a thanksgiving service in the church they attended. Lots of people wanted to speak in that, and the same was true of the service held in the hospital where Derek had been training. 'Getting through' these occasions was emotionally draining, but both Derek and Mary were relieved that they were able to do so without weeping in public.

Afterwards

After the funeral there is often a sense of anti-climax. And as time goes by, the challenges of coping with sudden death change. They come in waves, and some, such as those during anniversaries, Christmas and New Year with special memories, can be predicted; others catch you unawares, occasioned by a place, a particular sound or smell, or a memory prompted by something you read or see on television or in a film. The first anniversary of the death can be particularly difficult: in Michael's case it was marked by planting a tree in his memory in the city where he had been studying, an event organised by his friends and colleagues. Some people send cards on the anniversary, which can be a mixed blessing – 'fine if it helps them, but...' was Mary's comment. The risk is that the scar tissue which is beginning to grow is broken and the painful wound again exposed.

Why?

And what of the inevitable question – why? Initially, the numbness of shock meant that Derek and Mary felt they had nothing intelligent they could say; no rationalisation they could offer. As time went on, Derek still did not feel he wanted to ask the question why. 'God chooses when we go; He is in charge and He had taken Michael early.' Mary felt she had a choice: to be bitter and twisted or to accept what had happened and move on. 'We cannot live in the past, in the "what might have been."' Both were conscious of the needs of their other children. Michael's brother, who was 18 at the time of Michael's death, did not want to talk to Michael's friends about it until several years after the event. Time heals – but can life ever be the same again?

A fatal step

Elisabeth was a much-loved and respected teacher. With her husband William, they led a house-group in their local church and offered generous, and much appreciated hospitality to students at the nearby university. When Elisabeth retired, she, William and one of their daughters went away for a celebratory weekend at a south coast resort. Walking out on the harbour wall, Elisabeth paused and looked up at a helicopter overhead. To get a better view she stepped backwards, slipped and fell onto the rocks below. Within the hour she had died.

It was by any reckoning a devastating blow. Yet Elisabeth's funeral was a celebration of her life and gifts as a teacher, a mother, a hostess and a Christian leader, and a deep expression of care and sympathy for William, and their children and grandchildren. No-one could even begin to address that nagging question why – but in the funeral sermon the congregation was reminded that this event underlined the brutal fact that we simply do not know when death will come. And therefore, we should be ready for it, as Elisabeth was, and her family knew she was.

Dying alone

Sylvia had had to retire early from teaching because of ill health. Being unmarried she lived on her own but had a large number of friends, not to mention godchildren, and once free from the pressures of school, was able to live a normal life. One weekend, her friends could not contact her at home. After repeated attempts the police were called and entered her flat to find her dead from – it was later revealed at the inquest – an allergic reaction to some food she had eaten at an evening out. She had been alone when she died. Her many friends and her sister and nephew were devastated. It was so sudden, so unexpected, so undeserved.

For Sylvia death came suddenly. Happily, she was ready – she was a Christian. And she knew too the pain of bereavement. After her own mother's death she had written: 'So what can I say? God is good all the time – all the time God is good. He has done everything well'. Those words were not written lightly. She added, 'I miss Mum so much and sometimes the pain of loss is almost physical.' Her experience of suffering and deep disappointment in her own life, even before her mother's death, equipped Sylvia with a deep sensitivity to the needs of others which shone through both in her career as a teacher and in her care for other people, particularly children. Though she died alone, her funeral was a celebration of a deeply appreciated teacher, colleague, and friend whose life of care and service had been suddenly cut short.

A biking accident – and guilt

Peter, a bachelor in his early twenties, loved his motor bike and enjoyed going out in the evening with his friends. His parents, and particularly his mother, tried not to worry about him getting back late but, after several occasions when he was later than normal, his mother asked him to try to come home earlier so that they did not have to wait up too long for him.

The knock on the door did not bring good news. The policeman told Peter's distraught mother that he had been involved in an accident and was unconscious in hospital and very seriously ill. A few days later he died without regaining consciousness. From that day on, his mother blamed herself: if only, she said, she had not badgered him about being late, the accident might not have occurred. For many years after she lovingly tended his grave, but sadly from the day of his funeral she could not bring herself to attend church again.

No time to prepare

In all the instances recounted above neither the person who died nor their relatives and friends had time to prepare. Earlier generations in our culture were more familiar with sudden death, whether from disease, accident or war. My parents' generation were only too familiar with the sight of the telegram boy bringing the dreaded news of a husband, a father or a son who had been killed in action in the world wars. In mining communities, and amongst those whose livelihoods depended upon the sea, the possibility of tragic accidents was ever present. Few would actually talk about it but the possibility was always there in the background.

In the current era, with – thankfully – limited wars, and significant advances in medicine and health and safety procedures, the incidence of sudden death is rarer, and death and dying are sidelined from our conversations, if not from our thinking. We expect that governments and the medical professions will be able to extend life expectancy, and adjust our life-styles accordingly. In consequence, we do not think or talk about dying, and when we are confronted with it we find coping all the more difficult. To address this deficit in our thinking and our talking is, of course, the main purpose of this book.

The shared experience

When, as in the instances related above, we have to deal with the fact of the sudden death of someone we know and love, it is helpful to know that others have been this way before and that we can draw some reassurance from hearing of their experience: the initial numbness, the sense of bewilderment and the inner aching pain; the struggle between the desire to be alone with one's grief and the need for comfort, consolation and practical help to get through even today; the need, in the midst of one's own pain and grief, to provide comfort and support to other members of the family, particularly children; the added complications of the 'formalities' which have to be undergone, particularly if there is an inquest or press interest; the weariness at having yet again to explain what has happened to those who have not yet heard; and, after the immediate furore, that aching gap in one's life and the awareness of the need, the desire, somehow to recover positive memories of the one we have lost. Life must, and will, go on. It cannot be the same but it need not be without hope. We will say more about this in later chapters.

Notes
[1] *A Song for Jenny,* BBC2, 9 July, 2015
[2] Names and some details changed to ensure anonymity.

6

SUICIDE

Elaine Sugden

The intentional taking of one's life is a tragic event, an act of despair. Suicide is a desperate attempt to escape suffering that has become unbearable. You can't make a person suicidal by showing that you care. Talking with a potential victim can make a difference. Talking with a bereaved survivor is essential.

Talking about the possibility of suicide is important

'Most people who commit suicide don't want to die – they just want to stop hurting.'

Harvard Health Publications [1]

Engaging with someone who is severely depressed and/or talking about death can be very worthwhile.

The evidence suggests that bringing up the subject of suicide and discussing it openly is one of the most helpful things you can do, and can be a relief to the person concerned.[2] A way of doing this could be with a sympathetic question: 'Have you ever thought of ending it all?' or, 'Are you having thoughts of suicide?' You are not putting ideas in their head, you are showing that you are concerned, that you take them seriously, and that it's OK for them to share their pain with you.

Be calm and non-judgmental; reassure the person that there is help. Encourage the person to tell their doctor, a therapist, or another adult they trust. Sometimes it might be necessary for you to inform helpful authorities. (See NHS choices website below). For this reason, it is important not to let yourself be sworn to secrecy.

People do better with good friends with whom they can share their anxieties and despair. It is good to talk.

Some will prefer to talk to The Samaritans: 'People talk to us anytime they like, in their own way, and off the record – about whatever's getting to them. You don't have to be suicidal.'[3]

But many people who commit suicide give no warning to anyone that they are thinking about it. They know that if they are to be successful, they must keep their plans to themselves.

The Harvard Medical School website[4] gives this helpful list of things that can put an individual at a higher risk for suicide in the short term:

- an episode of depression, psychosis or anxiety
- a significant loss, such as the death of a partner or the loss of a job
- a personal crisis or life stress, especially one that increases a sense of isolation or leads to a loss of self-esteem, such as a breakup or divorce
- loss of social support, for example, because of a move or when a close friend relocates
- an illness or medication that triggers a change in mood

But the website goes on to say: 'We all face crises or problems like these. One difference is that among individuals who take their own lives, these situations cause such pain or hopelessness they can't see any other way out.'[4]

Suicide is not uncommon

Every 85 minutes in the UK, someone dies from suicide. In 2013, 6708 suicides were recorded in UK and Ireland.[5] In 2013, suicide was the leading cause of death in England and Wales for men aged between 20 and 49 years of age. The highest suicide rate was in men in the 45 to 59-year age range. The incidence in men was over three times more than that in women.[6] The highest incidence was in those with mental health problems and, particularly, in the first few months after diagnosis. Admission to hospital, intended to provide a safe environment, might reduce but does not eliminate the risk.

> 'One characteristic that emerges in almost all studies is a desperate sense of hopelessness in the suicidal. The hopelessness may puzzle and distress friends and family as inexplicable – but is nonetheless dark, black, painful and (in the end) unendurable in the sufferer.'
>
> Mike Parsons, 'Suicide and the Church'[7]

Efforts to reduce the risk

Most suicide attempts are planned within an hour of the event, so that removal of obvious methods would seem sensible. Nationally, the removal of coal gas, carbon monoxide from car exhausts and paracetamol sold in large quantities did result in a drop in incidence of suicide by each of these means, though substitution by other methods has occurred.[8]

Antidepressants in those with known depression and suicidal thoughts can be useful, but some of those depressed are fearful of taking antidepressants, whilst a significant proportion stop taking medication some time before taking their own life.

The bereaved survivors

For each of the over 6000 people who took their own life in 2013, there was at least one and often several bereft survivors.

One such survivor, S, tells the story of the youngest of his three brothers who was in his early fifties when, over fifteen years ago, he took his own life. This brother had a challenging childhood illness which was kept secret outside the family. He developed into a passionate and deeply sensitive person, ever eager to help those around him. After leaving school, he did a few different jobs and then joined the family business, which deteriorated and closed down when his father retired. He married and later adopted three children with a history of abuse and who, in their late teens got into various scrapes with the police. He and his wife took on another business, which failed, and they separated.

Latterly, he partnered a single mother with three children. Against legal advice, he bought a house in their joint names a few months before this relationship failed. He realised she had been deceiving him and that he had lost much of his money; feeling that he had made a mess of things he committed a carefully planned suicide, leaving letters to his lover, his adult children and others. His instructions for a service of remembrance celebrated the Christian faith he had never left.

This is what the bereaved brother S wrote recently: 'To begin with I thought I *will* find out all that had happened; I will uncover the truth. But quickly we realised it was impossible to know all the circumstances. Some good friends of his wrote a detailed and helpful account of their dealings with him in his last few months. But there were large areas of obscurity. Our parents were sad but did not want to hear unwelcome detail; our mother preferred to think he had died of natural causes, despite clear evidence to the contrary.

We could have held a family conference with some of his friends to try to learn more. But we all knew different bits of the story.'

The question 'Why?' is on the lips and in the minds of family, friends and acquaintances after every death by suicide.

'They have forced their goodbye on you, a goodbye you have not wanted and cannot now undo. For that, you have only the ringing, unanswerable whys.'[9]

The most common overriding emotion for those left behind is guilt. 'If only I had – noticed something was wrong/ been there/not said those cross words....' Guilt under these circumstances is almost always unjustified, but acutely felt.

'I wonder if I should have said something. He mentioned a while before he died that he was having a hard time and I didn't tell anyone, maybe I should have. Maybe he would still be alive if I'd said something. People say it wasn't my fault but I can't help thinking I should have been able to help him.'

Sister of 18-year-old[10]

Some are angry at, or feel rejected by, the one who took their own life. Blame is common: God, the employer, the other parent. Those who find themselves in the firing line need to soak up the anger and blame rather than retaliate. The bereaved are hurting deeply. They need someone to talk to, who will listen to them and who will try to understand what they might be feeling. They need friends and perhaps to be directed to some useful resources.

Ben, just short of 20 years, had been troubled with schizophrenia for almost four years, during which he had self-harmed. He was thought to be doing rather better when he went out on a bike ride and didn't return. His parents told me:

'The presence of people was helpful, just being there, listening, whether to speech or in silence holding hands. (It would be OK to ask the suffering person whether or not they want you to stay). We didn't feel they were intruding but were glad to have interest and care. Don't be frightened of tears either in yourself or the one/s you are trying to express care for. Be prepared to weep with them.'

Men and women often react differently, but it is important to allow grief to be expressed.

Hector was 21 when, in 2011, he took his own life. His father, from experience, said: 'Wives and partners often wish for men to be in touch with their feminine side so that they understand how they feel. But the minute a man bursts into tears and appears to "lose control" or be less of a man, they are truly shocked and don't really like it.'

Jamie Doward, *The Observer News*, 1.11.15

Bereavement after suicide is long-term and you will not be able to 'fix' it or make it go away. People need assistance and support, usually for a long period of time, as they come to terms with what has happened.

'I was in deep shock after his suicide even though I had been bracing for it. He'd attempted it four times, so I guess I thought he wasn't really ever going to die, that it would be OK.'[11]

Talking and practical help

Some more thoughts from S (in the story above) about his brother's death by suicide:

'There is sometimes a kindness in silence, perhaps particularly after a suicide. How much do we really ever know even about those closest to us? We did of course share memories, photos, and mementos; still on his birthday we talk about our dear departed brother. There is certainly comfort in such sharing.

'Any life cut short by illness or accident causes distress. But suicide aggravates and intensifies such feelings. However, much comfort can be derived from the sympathy and practical support of friends, relatives, colleagues, neighbours and others, especially when this is given unconditionally, without prying or gossip or curiosity. And those who knew my brother were often ready to speak of his many excellent and lovable qualities.'

See also chapter 8 *Talking to Children* and chapter 13 *How We Can Help*.

Notes

[1] Harvard Health Publications, Harvard medical school: www.helpguide.org/articles/suicide-prevention/suicide-prevention-helping-someone-who-is-suicidal.htm

[2] See: www.helpguide.org/home-pages/suicide-prevention.htm

[3] The Samaritans web site: www.samaritans.org

[4] Harvard medical school, Harvard Health Publications: www.helpguide.org/articles/suicide-prevention/suicide-prevention-helping-someone-who-is-suicidal.htm

[5] The Samaritans statistical report: www.samaritans.org/sites/default/files/kcfinder/branches/branch-96/files/Suicide_statistics_report_2015.pdf

[6] Office for National Statistics http://webarchive.nationalarchives.gov.uk/20160105160709/http://www.ons.gov.uk/ons/dcp171778_395145.pdf

[7] Mike Parsons, 'Suicide and the Church', Grove pastoral series, p123

[8] Sarchiapone, Marco, et al., 'Controlling Access to Suicide Means', Int J Environ Res Public Health (2011); 8(12): 4550–4562; and Kreitman, Norman, 'The coal gas story. United Kingdom suicide rates, 1960-71', Brit. J. Prev. Soc. Med (1976) 30:86-93.

[9] www.christianitytoday.com/women/2012/august/in-wake-of-suicides-silence-why-blame-is-never-answer.html

[10] Support after Suicide: www.supportaftersuicide.org.au/

[11] Allan's story, Suicide support website.

Other resources

NHS choices suicide warning: www.nhs.uk/Conditions/Suicide/Pages/warning-signs.aspx

Wertheimer, Alison, *A Special Scar: the experience of people bereaved by suicide* (Routledge, 1991)

7

THE DEATH OF A BABY

Elaine Sugden

Miscarriage, stillbirth and neonatal death

Parents develop a relationship with a child from the beginning of pregnancy, long before birth, and so a dead baby produces enormous shock and ongoing grief. There is profound sadness at the loss of expectations for the future.

Early miscarriage is common, late miscarriage, stillbirth and neonatal death less so, but many of us will know family or friends who have experienced these events, and some will want to know what happens around this time. As with all the situations in this book, we firmly believe it is good to talk (and more importantly listen) to the bereaved parents, as well as to one another about this event which has too often been treated without due consideration of the loss.

The three stages of pregnancy

Doctors divide pregnancy into three stages called 'trimesters'. The times are calculated from the end of the mother's last period.

The first trimester is up to 13 weeks of pregnancy.
The second trimester is from 14-24 weeks of pregnancy.
The third and final trimester starts from 25 weeks of pregnancy.

Miscarriage

This is when a baby dies before 24 weeks of pregnancy. About 1 in 5 pregnancies ends before 24 weeks. This is called a miscarriage, rather than stillbirth, as 24 weeks is the legal age at which a baby is thought to stand a good chance of survival.

Early miscarriage – when a baby dies up to 12 weeks of pregnancy. Early miscarriage is common and sometimes happens before even the mother herself is aware of the pregnancy.

Late miscarriage – when a baby dies between 14 and 24 weeks of pregnancy. Late miscarriage is less common.

Will there be a birth or death certificate after a miscarriage?

After miscarriage, whether early or late, the law does not require a certificate.

Although there is no legal certificate after a pregnancy loss before 24 weeks, some hospitals do provide a certificate for parents to mark what has happened. For many parents this is an important memento.

The Miscarriage Association (MA) has suggestions of how to obtain a certificate if you have not been given one, but would like to have one. Their website details are below.

After a late miscarriage, most hospitals offer a simple funeral and either burial or cremation. Some hospitals offer this for all babies, no matter how early the loss and whether or not there is a fully formed body. Hospital practice is improving all the time but sadly not all hospitals treat the remains of an early loss with the respect needed.

What happens to the baby after a miscarriage?

'I initially declined to hold my baby I was so scared to see how he might look. But a few hours later I changed my mind and a very kind midwife brought him back into the room. I was pleased I had seen my baby who was tiny but perfectly formed.'

Mother after a late miscarriage, MA website

There is no law about what should happen to the body of a miscarried baby.

Stillbirth

This is when a baby is born dead at or after 24 weeks of pregnancy. Stillbirth is uncommon but unfortunately, it is not rare. In the UK about one baby in 200 is stillborn.

Holding your stillborn baby

Many parents decide to see and hold their baby after the birth, and nearly all find it helpful. Some do not and this is an individual decision, with no right or wrong way to respond. Sometimes one parent makes a different decision from the other. Both parents need time to think what is best for them.

Should there be a postmortem?

When doctors are unsure about the cause of death, they might ask the parents to consider a postmortem examination and other tests to help to find out. This will only be done with their agreement and written consent.

When the results are available the doctor should arrange to go through these with the parents. More than half the time the cause of death is not found.

Saying goodbye

The parents can decide to say goodbye to the baby either before or after the postmortem.

A certification and registering of a stillbirth

The doctor or midwife will give a certificate of stillbirth. The stillbirth should be registered within the time given on the UK Government (UK Gov) website below.

Will there be a funeral?

The bodies of babies who are stillborn (that is, born dead after 24 weeks of pregnancy), or who are born alive but then die, must by law be buried or cremated.

Neonatal Death

A neonatal death is when a baby is born alive but dies within the first 28 days of life. Premature birth, congenital abnormality and infection are the main causes. Whatever the cause, a baby has died and it is a hugely sad time. The death must be registered, the doctors might ask permission from the parent/s for a postmortem examination and burial or cremation will need to be arranged. (See chapter 12: *Practical Matters*.)

Sudden Unexpected Death in Infancy

The sudden loss of a seemingly perfect baby, who increasingly became a part of the family as each day went past, is devastating for the parents and those who love them.

'Sudden Infant Death' is the term used to describe the sudden and unexpected death of a baby that is initially unexplained. The usual medical term is 'Sudden Unexpected Death in Infancy' (SUDI) or, if the baby was over 12 months old, Sudden Unexpected Death in Childhood (SUDC). In spite of following advice on how to reduce the risk of sudden infant death, it can still happen.

> 'Parents are shocked, bewildered, and distressed. Parents who are innocent of blame in their child's death often feel responsible nonetheless and imagine ways in which they might have contributed to or prevented the tragedy.'
>
> *Paediatrics*, Feb 2001

As well as shock, there is bound to be a feeling of guilt – how could I have prevented it? Although there will be a postmortem, in at least half of cases no cause at all is found.

At the time of death, there will be routine questions from medical and judicial teams, which, depending how they are said, can seem intrusive and accusatory. (It is important that the small proportion of deaths where there has been malpractice can be detected.) Only after a thorough death scene investigation, postmortem examination and review of case records, can a diagnosis of sudden unexpected death be given as the cause of death.

These procedures might give a reason why the infant died, and how other children in the family, including children born later, might be affected.

For the parents of the approximately 300 sudden and unexpected infant deaths which occur in the UK each year, it is an enormous shock and an event which will have an effect on them for the rest of their lives. How doctors and others deal with them after the death can also have a deep and lasting effect.

How can family and friends help?

In all the situations described in this chapter, it is important for us to remember that no baby can be replaced.

Family and friends need to be aware of the acute and ongoing pain and loss felt by the parents. Listen rather than talk, send cards and flowers, leave messages, offer specific help. (See chapter 13: *How we can help*)

'Nobody talks about it, the topic is completely avoided or worse, I am avoided. To me, I lost our baby, the baby who already had its own room and crib, we were thinking about names and how childcare would work. No one seems to acknowledge what has happened. Talk to your friends/ family who have gone through a miscarriage, ask them if they want to talk about it. Sometimes you just need a hug, sometimes you want to get it all out and have a long talk, no responses needed just acknowledgment and comfort.'

Posted by a mum, a month after a miscarriage.

**Sources for miscarriage, stillbirth
and sudden death of a baby**

Miscarriage Association (MA):
www.miscarriageassociation.org.uk

Babycentre general:
www.babycentre.co.uk/a1014800/when-a-baby-is-stillborn

Babycentre website on how friends can help
www.babycentre.co.uk/x1014809/my-friends-have-
recently-lost-their-baby-is-there-anything-i-can-say-or-do-
to-help-them

UK Government site https://www.gov.uk/register-stillbirth
giving information about registering a stillbirth. At the time
of writing this must be done within 21 days in Scotland, 42
days in England and one year in N Ireland.

SANDS Stillbirth and neonatal death charity:
www.uk-sands.org

Babyloss gives information about other support agencies
www.babyloss.com/index.php

The Lullaby Trust offers confidential support to anyone
affected by the sudden and unexpected death of a baby or
young toddler. www.lullabytrust.org.uk

8

TALKING TO CHILDREN

Elaine Sugden

Children and death[1]

Much as we would like to, we cannot protect children from death. Children themselves die and parents of dependent children die. Both events are indescribably sad. Different families will do things differently, but we hope that this chapter, together with some of the suggested resources, will be useful to anyone trying to cope with or to help in this difficult situation.

It is important at the outset to use the words 'death' or 'died'. Words or phrases like 'lost' or 'passed away' can be confusing for children. If someone is 'lost', why isn't anybody looking for him/her?

This chapter will look firstly at children's early experiences of death and the maturing understanding of teenagers, followed by experiences of the death of a parent, brother or sister and then of a child's own death.

The Death of a Pet

Children, like adults, need to understand that death is a natural part of life. The death of a pet is often a child's first introduction to the loss and grief of death. Pets can die after an illness, suddenly after an accident or with general failure as they become very old. Although the pet might look to be asleep there are no signs of life; the pet is dead.

Young children often ask a lot of questions. It is important to listen carefully and think how to respond in a simple, straightforward way. What is said and how, together with support for the child, as the pet is spoken about lovingly and with good memories, will help. It will also give the child a way to relate to others who have had a similar experience. Children copy the behaviour of adults.

General understanding of death in childhood

Children's understanding of the death of a person changes at different ages. A pre-school child might not understand the word 'death' and might continue to expect the person to return. It is not unusual for a child to think they can get the person back, particularly if they do something special or perhaps just 'be good'. We should always try to answer their questions truthfully; short, honest explanations are the best. It is not wrong to say 'I don't know' when that is true.

There isn't a perfect way or the perfect words to say. What matters is that what is said comes from the heart, with honesty and love.

'I told my little boy that people die when their bodies really don't work very well any more, that they are very, very ill and that then it is the right time to die.' (Quote from a mother of a 3-year-old who asked, 'Why do people die?' and, 'When will I die?' This 3-year-old boy had a 5-year-old brother who was very ill and died a few months after this.)[2]

By the ages of 6 or 7, magic and myths are important ideas, children are curious and imaginative. They might start to talk about heaven, paradise and an after-life. They will link a death to what they know and begin to realise the finality of death.

> When told of the death of their great grandmother, my cousin's children were then aged 6 and 5. One asked: 'Who shot her?' and the other: 'Did she go to heaven in a rocket?'

This is the age when children start to feel responsible. They must be reassured that the death of a person special to them is not their fault and that it is okay to enjoy themselves.

Understanding develops during childhood and usually, by the age of 10 or 12, children understand the finality of death.

Not all children will have talked about death with their families before someone special and loved dies. They need to know that whatever happens there will always be someone to take care of them.

Some children don't want to talk and don't ask questions, but those caring for them – parent, teachers and others, might see changes in behaviour.

Teenagers

Teenagers have an adult understanding that death means the end of life and body, but not how to cope with it. They are becoming independent from parents and may consider themselves indestructible. Self and body image are important and they will have ideas about the spiritual aspects of life and death. The reality of death challenges their ideas of themselves. Some teenagers are very emotional; some want to talk and ask questions whilst others prefer to find help from friends rather than from family. Some need to be alone. Feelings go up and down; guilt, anger, loss, can lead to reckless behaviour, such as fighting, drug or alcohol abuse or sexual promiscuity. School avoidance or poor performance at this stage is common.

Teenagers, like adults and children, need to be listened to

and given the opportunity to ask questions, tell their stories and share their grief. They may look like adults, but they are not yet adults. They are not in a position to 'be strong' or 'grown up', or to 'care for the family' as they are often encouraged to do. They need time to mourn and grieve. Caring adults can help teenagers cope with their grief, which is a natural expression of love for the person who died. It is all right to be sad and to have lots of different feelings, but expectations for good behaviour should be maintained. Exercise, music, art or other activities might be unexpectedly useful, and doing things, like playing games together, can give opportunities for questions and conversations. A peer support group can be very helpful. Professional help is sometimes needed when grief and its outworking are producing serious and unsettling consequences.

Spiritual understanding of death

For many children this will be affected not only by age but by the religion and beliefs of their parents. The children's bereavement charity Winston's Wish suggests the following: It may be best to say something like: 'People have all sorts of beliefs about what happens after someone dies. We know that they can't come back and visit us or ring on the phone. Being dead isn't like being in another country. These are some of the things that people believe – and I believe this.... I wonder what you believe? You may change what you believe as you grow older.'[3]

The Death of a Parent (or main carer)

Each day in the UK more than 100 children lose a parent.[4]

One of the saddest events is the death of a parent of a dependent child. I remember a mother with imminently terminal cancer who came to my clinic. Her husband described how just that morning they had told their two young children that mummy was soon going to die. We shed tears together. At that time, I too had young children.

When the parent is dying

Those who work with children whose parent is dying emphasise that it is important for children's lives and routines to be kept as normal as possible. Time with the parent is also important, and for them to be allowed to help care for mum or dad. However, it is also important that the child is not the main carer. Help must be appropriate to the age of the child; children must be allowed to be children. Older children can helpfully be kept informed about how the illness is progressing, and what is happening to the parent. Those dealing with children who have experienced the death of a parent say that such involvement helps the child later on in bereavement. Keeping children (of whatever age) away, although done with the best intentions, has been found to be less helpful.

School

Children benefit from continuing to go to school. School keeps at least part of normal life, and older children can find friends a source of strength. But the school should be informed about the situation so that teachers and other staff can be aware of the reason for any changes in behaviour.

> 'He was very distracted in class. I had no idea his mother had died. He never told us and I never thought to ask.'
>
> A teacher, in *Beyond the Rough Rock*[5]

After the death of a parent or parent figure

The decision as to whether or not the child sees the body after death will depend on the other parent or main carer and, most importantly, on the wishes of the child. It can be helpful for a child to see the parent's body (which will usually be in the care of the funeral director) but someone they trust should prepare them for what will happen: who will be there and what they will see. They need to know that the body will be cold, because it is not working and that it cannot feel pain anymore; imagination is less easy to manage than reality. It is often better to see that the parent they love has left the body because it is no longer needed. Soon the body will be buried or burned.[6]

It might be necessary to change this advice somewhat if the body is mutilated, but even then it might be possible to see part of the body.

> 'My body is just my reflection – when you die you leave your reflection. Your real self leaves your body and goes into another world' – said by an 11-year-old boy a year before he died.[7]

Children, like adults, will vary in their wish to visit a grave. Some want to be there soon and often, whilst others might take many months or never want to visit. Try to leave the opportunity open, but do not force.

Ongoing concerns

Children are often worried that they, or another special person in their life, might die soon. Although unlikely, it can happen. As always, it is important to listen and take their concerns seriously. Reassurance that they will always be loved and cared for is important.

You or the child might fear that details of the one who has

died will be forgotten. Talk about the person, build and save memories of special times they enjoyed with that special person. Cry together.

Don't forget: children and adults usually like to talk about the special person who has died, long after the death. They want to keep remembering the person and what he/she meant to them and others. The death anniversary is a special opportunity for remembering.

Death of a parent or main carer from suicide

Winston's Wish, the bereavement charity for children, notes that 1 in every 10 children they work with has had a parent die from suicide. Each year around 6000 families are bereaved by suicide.[8]

It is difficult to talk to adults about suicide and, usually, even more difficult to talk to children, though often children understand more than adults think they do. Not telling the truth and having family secrets can bring extra problems later on.

Joe was a young teenager when his mother disappeared and later was found dead. As an adult, Joe said: 'It was not spoken of, never discussed in the family at all, I cannot remember ever having a conversation with my father about it. That was the way the family coped. I felt that I was to blame. I think I've spent a lot of my life trying to make up for it. My last memory of her was of her being very angry with me. I can't remember what I had done.'[9]

The most usual question after a suicide for both children and adults is 'Why?' Even if a note has been left, the question remains. Everyone connected to the person only has part of the picture.

The most usual reaction of a child or adult to the suicide of someone close to them is guilt and the feeling that they are in some way responsible or that they might have been able to prevent it. Also, the family can feel there is a stigma, which adds to their bereavement burden.

Children in this position often have questions to ask and a story to tell. It is important that they are given the opportunity to talk. Once again, honesty is the best policy and it is best for children to be given simple but truthful information. They need someone to listen to how they are feeling and give them strong reassurance that it is not their fault, and that they will be loved and cared for.

The Death of a Brother or Sister

Might this happen to me?
When a brother or sister is very ill, dying or has died, it is very common for brothers and sisters to worry that they too might fall ill and die. They need any questions to be answered honestly and simply, and they need a great deal of love and reassurance. It might be very difficult for this to come from grieving parents. This is when a trusted and loved relative or friend can have an important role.

Feeling left out
There can also be understandable concern about all the attention being given to the one who is ill. After death, there can be the idea that the child who has died was the favourite. It is not unusual for parents to give all care and attention to the sick child, feeling that they can make up to their other child/children later on. Sadly, this does not seem to work well. Children need day-to-day assurance that they are loved

and cared about just as much as the ill child. Even young children are aware when things are difficult for the family, and that a brother or sister is very ill and needs special care. If it is impossible for the parents to do so, it is helpful for someone to be there to answer questions and give undivided attention to children who themselves are very worried about their ill brother or sister.

Let them be involved

Those who have dealt many times with this situation in the capacity of a nurse, social worker or teacher, advise that it is best for children to be involved in some way with the care of a dying sibling. Even though this is the professional view, which should be shared gently and with support, parents know their children best and their decisions must be respected. Wherever possible, it is also good for brothers and sisters to play and do other normal things together.

The death of a child

The death of a child in the UK is uncommon, but even so, around 5,000 children between birth and 19 years die each year. Around two-thirds of those deaths happen in the first year of life. Different causes are more common at different ages, but after the first year, injuries, poisoning and cancer contribute significantly.[10]

For the families of these children, statistics are irrelevant; their child dies. No two deaths are the same. Some deaths are sudden, and without time for any sort of preparation. Others have a longer illness or disability during which some grieving often starts to happen.

Although I have used information from several sources as well as from my own experience, I would thoroughly recommend a booklet called 'Facing the Death of Your Child'. It is available now to read online or download.[11]

Talking to a child who is expected to die

It is an individual decision for a parent of a dying child if, when and how to talk to their child about dying. The parent lives on after the child's death, and it is important that they feel they have had control and done what felt right for them. Some parents want to make preparation for death and a funeral whilst the child is alive but many don't want to.

Teenagers in particular sometimes want to 'have a say' about what will happen at their funeral.

All but two parents in an interview study of 13 children (ages 8-17) with life threatening illness, wanted to be in charge of what their children understood and were told about their illness. Some children, younger and older, felt they wanted to hear directly from the medical staff about their illness and response to treatment; others were happy to learn everything from their parents.[12]

Children can be involved in decisions about their own treatment. Parents must sign the consent form, but whenever possible, children should agree.

'It's better if they tell you most things because most people like to know what's wrong. I know I did.'

Quote from boy with cancer, aged 10.[13]

Deciding not to talk

It is understandable that some parents in this situation make the decision not to talk to their child about death. Sometimes, parents make every effort to make sure that neither they, nor anyone else speaks to their child about dying. They fear that they, as well as the sick child, will 'lose hope'. This can be particularly difficult with older children and teenagers who realise they are not responding to treatment. They spend time talking with friends and probably know they are going to die, but also know that the parent does not want to discuss this.

Some parents always intend to tell 'when I need to' or 'when the time is right' or 'sometime'. However, when questions have not been answered honestly from the time of diagnosis, it can be difficult to change the approach.

> 'Our daughter was only 10 and we decided not to tell her. The doctor said from her experience it was best to tell – I wanted to but we just couldn't tell her.'
>
> Quote from mother whose daughter had a new cancer diagnosis [14]

Sometimes, parents do want to discuss and give their child every opportunity but their child does not want to talk to them, though might talk to a brother, sister or friend.

> 'Be Honest. Ultimately honesty is probably the best policy but the presentation of truth will differ from child to child and family to family.'
>
> A senior children's cancer specialist [15]

Children's Questions

Most children, whatever their age, ask questions, though sometimes not many. Questions are a good way of knowing when a child is ready to listen, as well as what they want to know (this also works with adults).

'My lovely daughter actually wrote on a piece of paper, "Am I dying?" She couldn't talk but I could explain to her. I said, "Yes, we think you are not going to get better this time and that you will die." I couldn't believe it when she actually wrote back, "Thanks for telling me, that's what I thought too."'

Mother of a 16-year-old girl[16]

This task of answering questions honestly is not easy, but very worthwhile. It is probably easier if done from the start of a difficult diagnosis. 'Kids can cope' in a way we do not imagine they can.

Children and teenagers often know that they are seriously ill whether or not they have been told. They might have guessed, overheard someone talking or had a dream.

Consider asking for help

It is not easy to talk to your child when there is a serious diagnosis, and if you are in this situation, you might need help. Be prepared to ask for help from medical and nursing staff, social workers or play specialists, especially if you know that someone seems to have a special relationship with your child.

Families find they grow closer when they are honest with one another, rather than avoiding painful issues. The opportunity might be lost for parents and children to voice their love for one another, to cry together or for a child or teenager to say what they would like to do before they die, or even what should happen at their funeral. Parents continue to be surprised by the maturity of their children and what they are thinking.

Information Step by step

The information might need to be given over a period of time, answering questions honestly and straightforwardly.

> 'My brave, brave son asked me, "Am I getting better, cos the chemo has been stopped?" I told him, "We have stopped the chemo, because it is not working any more...." A few days later he asked me, "Does that mean I could die?" and, together, his mother and I sat down and told him, "Yes, you could." I never want to go through that talk again. I thought I was going to be sick. Again, a few days later he came and asked a bit more. It taught me how he really needed only a tiny bit of information a bit at a time. It made it much easier for all of us, in a sad kind of way.'
>
> Father of a 10-year-old boy[17]

How will my family cope?

Children's major concern in this situation is often for their parents and how they will cope without them. Dying children are less distressed when the family share their grief and show love to one another, as well as to their suffering child. Sometimes, the dying child 'hangs on' to life because of worries about how mum and/or dad will cope. They need to be reassured that it is alright to 'let go' and that all the special people: mum, dad, brothers, sisters and others will be OK because they will continue to love and support one another.

Medical decisions

It is not possible to save every child's life. Sadly, the time comes when a child's illness is no longer responding to treatment and the child is almost certainly going to die.

Doctors, parents and, where appropriate, older children, agree together that treatment against the disease is not working and that the main task now is to make sure that remaining life (and death) are as comfortable as possible.

Sometimes parents or the wider family are unable to accept this plan, and decide to take their child overseas for the promise of 'more successful' treatment. The media makes much of these cases, especially where fund raising has been involved. We tend not to hear of the later, inevitable, deaths of these children.

The time comes when there is a move from active treatment and investigations to what is called 'palliative care', which involves the management of pain and other symptoms. Children's hospices can play an important part in helping families to cope in this situation. Some families want their child to die in the hospice or in hospital, but more usually, the child will die at home. Either way, they will die surrounded by their loving family.

The sudden death of a child
In the situation of the sudden death of a child, there is no time for these decisions. Parents are thrown into bereavement and need deep understanding and care from family, friends, the secular and faith communities, as well as the medical profession. Many have also found help from local or national support organisations, some of which are listed at the end of this chapter.

In the UK in 2014[18]

2,129 children and young people died between the ages of 1 and 19 – that is around 6 children and young people per day.

2,013 babies died within 4 weeks of birth.

A further 911 babies died before reaching their first birthday.

This chapter has explored aspects of death involving children and has drawn widely on the experience of many. Even so, there will be more that others would want to add.

The key points of this chapter

- The understanding of death develops with the child
- Teenagers have an adult understanding that death means the end of life, but would not be expected to know how to cope with it
- Answering children's questions from the start honestly and with love is the best policy and draws the family together
- Children should not be the main carer for a dying parent, but usually find it helpful to be involved in caring in some way
- Children cope with their own early death better than we might fear
- Brothers and sisters should be involved, not excluded, and their daily need for attention and love supplied.

Notes

[1] I acknowledge invaluable help in the content and structure of this chapter, which I received from Sister Frances Dominica, Kathy Moore and Margot Shawyer. They generously shared their professional knowledge, advice and time. In addition, I drew heavily on a publication from the Children's Cancer and Leukaemia Group (CCLG) entitled 'Facing the Death of Your Child'. This gives some very general information about children and death, as well as detailed information for the parents of a dying child. With permission, I have used some of their stories.

[2] 'Facing the death of your child', CCLG publications, April 2015 www.cclg.org.uk/our-publications/bereavement/facing-the-death-of-your-child

[3] Winston's Wish website, 'Supporting You Talking About Death' www.winstonswish.org.uk/talking-about-death

[4] Winston's Wish website: About Us Facts and Figures

[5] Beyond the Rough Rock, Winston's Wish publications https://winstons-wish.myshopify.com/collections/books

[6] See *What Happens When Someone Dies: A book for adults and children to share together* (SeeSaw publication 2014) for helpful pictures of a funeral. www.seesaw.org.uk

[7] Sister Frances Dominica, 'Just My Reflection – helping parents do things their way when their child dies', www.helen&douglas house.org.uk

[8] Child Bereavement UK Why Are We Needed – statistics www.childbereavementuk.org

[9] Alison Wertheimer, *A Special Scar – The Experiences of People Bereaved by Suicide* (Routledge, 1992).

[10] 'Why Children Die: death in infants, children and young people in the UK', RCPCH report 1014 Woolf et al: www.ncb.org.uk/media/1130496/rcpch_ncb_may_2014_-_why_children_die_part_a.pdf

[11] www.cclg.org.uk/our-publications/bereavement/facing-the-death-of-your-child

[12] Young et el., BMJ 8.2.2003

[13] *British Medical Journal*, 8.2.2003, p305-308.

[14] Ibid.

[15] In *Children's Cancer and Leukaemia Group Contact Magazine*, Autumn 2003: www.cclg.org.uk/Contact-magazine

[16] Facing the death of your child, Children's Cancer and Leukaemia Group CCLG publications, April 2015: www.cclg.org.uk/our-publications/bereavement/facing-the-death-of-your-child

[17] Ibid.

[18] Child Bereavement UK, Why Are We Needed – see Note 8.

Other resources

www.rcpch.ac.uk/improving-child-health/child-mortality/child-mortality
Winston's Wish – Support, guidance and information from experienced professionals for anyone who is concerned about a child facing the death of a family member or who has already been bereaved.
Helpline and publications: www.winstonswish.org.uk
'As Big as it Gets: supporting a child when a parent is seriously ill', Winston's Wish 2012
'Beyond the Rough Rock: supporting a child who has been bereaved through suicide', Winston's Wish 2008

Other useful publications not specifically mentioned in the text:

Levine, Stephen, *Who Dies: An Investigation of Conscious Living and Conscious Dying*, (Gateway Books), chapter 9, 'Dying Children'. ISBN 0-946551-45-6
'Talking to Children and Teenagers when an Adult has Cancer', Macmillan Cancer Support 2016, edition 3
https://be.macmillan.org.uk/be/p-20644-talking-to-children-and-teenagers-when-an-adult-has-cancer.aspx

9

TALKING ABOUT LIFE AFTER DEATH

Martin Down

Different views

This could be the most important chapter in the book. One of the reasons why we do not talk about dying is that we are so unsure of what, if anything, comes after it. Doubt, confusion, fear – all fill our minds as we try to grapple with this question. Is there life after death? How can we know? How can we sort out all the ideas and beliefs that different people hold? Despair, at ever being able to find the answer, may lead us either to shrug our shoulders and give up trying, or to avoid asking the question in the first place. But if we have no hope that transcends death, then we will naturally be reluctant to think about it.

There is indeed such a vast range of ideas about life after death that we encounter today, that it seems very difficult to make any choice that is more than random, or wishful thinking.

Nothing

> To start with, whether we like it or not, we are all profoundly influenced by the scientific materialism of our Western world. Materialism denies the possibility of life after death at all: 'When you're dead, you're dead.'

If God exists, then this is not true.

On the other hand, most religions which include a belief in God in one form or another also include some sort of belief in life or existence after death, though the nature of these beliefs varies widely.

Eastern religions

The Eastern religions, such as Hinduism and Buddhism, believe in reincarnation. Some version of this belief has become quite common in the West, though usually in a somewhat crude and shallow form. The original idea was that souls have to ascend by degrees to a state of perfection, or reabsorption into the divine being. Each life that the soul lives, during these different incarnations, is a step up or down this ladder of perfection, depending on how well or how badly we have lived in this present life. The aim of life is to reach the point at which the soul achieves enlightenment or liberation and, therefore, does not need to go on being reincarnated. Then it merges like a drop of water into the ocean of being.

The clumsy version of this belief in Western culture is simply that at the end of one turn on the dodgems we climb into another car and go round again. Such a prospect of course is more or less appealing, depending on what sort of experience of life we have already had. Some people would be only too pleased not to have to live this life over again. It is also worth adding that in the Eastern religions, reincarnation is regarded as a punishment rather than a reward. We have to keep on enduring the sufferings of this life until our souls are purged.

Judaism, Christianity and Islam

These three religions all share some belief in life after death, though their understandings of this life, and of the qualifications for enjoying it, are different. It is fair to say that if most Western people retain any sort of belief in life after death, it is one that is derived from these faiths, in however muddled and partial a form. If the cards left with the bunches of flowers for those who have died are anything to go by, this popular faith consists of a belief that after we die we go to some place of peace and happiness, where our earthly cares and sufferings are over.

In the popular mind, not everyone qualifies for this reward: some people, like paedophiles and mass murderers, do not. In the popular mind, we ourselves, and our friends and neighbours, are good people, or good enough, and so we are heading for some sort of candy-floss existence on the other side. It must also be added that for the majority of people today the original emphasis in the world's religions on the over-riding importance of our relationship to God has been lost.

Tolerance

We live today in a society that prides itself on tolerance. We accept that people have different opinions and we do not like to challenge or argue with each other about them. Yet, for an opinion to deserve respect, there must be some evidence or reason to support it. And that is where the question of life after death seems to hit a brick wall. With good reason, people often justify their ignorance or unwillingness to talk about life after death with the comment that, 'How can we know what lies beyond death? No-one has ever come back to tell us.' But this is to ignore the resurrection of Jesus.

The resurrection of Jesus

Christians believe that someone has indeed come back from the dead: Jesus of Nazareth, a first century prophet of Israel, and, according to his followers more than a prophet, the Son of God. In his lifetime, Jesus said a great deal about life after death. His resurrection from the dead is proof for Christians that he knew what he was talking about.

The evidence for the resurrection of Jesus is spelt out in many books, such as those listed in the Resources section at the end of this chapter.

'Taking all the evidence together, it is not too much to say that there is no single historic incident better supported than the Resurrection of Christ.'

Brooke Foss Westcott, Bishop of Durham (1825-1901)

With the hard historical evidence supporting his resurrection from the dead, let us examine what Jesus says about life after death and the hope that he offers to those who will receive it. Like any other belief or opinion, each person must accept or reject this for themselves. In doing so, we must be sure that our decision is an informed and considered one. It may surprise us and take us way beyond our expectations.

Christian hope

This present world

Our common lot as human beings is to be born into a world not of our own making: a world of breathtaking grandeur and complexity, from the grandeur of the sun, the moon, the stars, of the mountains and the seas, to the complexity of all forms of life, including our own minds and bodies. It is a world of great beauty and goodness: a world of flowers and sunsets, of poetry and music, of love and friendship; but also a world of great ugliness and evil – a world of genocide and destruction, of lust and greed, of corruption and abuse.

We are born with both a great appetite for life, for the

opportunities and pleasures it offers us, and at the same time, a great fear of life, of the threats and sufferings that it may impose upon us, and above all, the fear of death and of the annihilation it may bring. The world presents us with a baffling mixture of good and evil, of beauty and ugliness, not only in the natural world but also in human behaviour.

God's purpose for us

The first thing to emphasise about the Christian hope is that it encompasses much more than life after death. It does indeed embrace individual survival, but it extends beyond that to the renewal of the whole creation. For the Christian, hope is not just a pious pipe-dream but an essential part of our understanding of God, and the world, as well as God's purposes for the world and for us. The Christian hope is that God, the designer and maker of the universe, is one day coming to put the world right, to clear up the mess that we have made of it, to do justice, destroy evil, and finally, create a new heaven and a new earth – a more perfect world in place of this one. The one through whom he will do all this is Jesus, the man whom he has sent to proclaim this good news and to initiate this work of redemption. Our confidence in this hope is based on Jesus' death and resurrection.

The Kingdom of God

The beginning of the message of Jesus is that the Kingdom of God is at hand. That means that this new order has already begun: that those who believe the Good News, who turn away from their old way of life and turn to God, can even now enjoy a foretaste of the life of the world to come, and are guaranteed to be part of that new world, when it is revealed in the fullness of time.

The miracles that Jesus performed, and which are still sometimes performed by his followers in his name, are signs of the power of God to right the things that have gone wrong, to cure suffering and disease, to conquer the forces of evil in the world, and to overcome the last enemy, which is death. A new life is already available to those who believe in and follow Jesus, and it is a life that will be eternal. What we have or have not done in the past need not be an obstacle to enjoying this new life, for in the Cross of Christ, God has forgiven and taken away our sins. Jesus has broken into this sad and suffering world that is heading for destruction, and the followers of Jesus are already on a journey that will take them out of this world and into the new world.

The life to come

In this present world, the followers of Jesus still experience suffering and the death of the body, but they do not despair or grieve over it as those who have no hope. In the New Testament, the Bible tells us that their bodies will sleep in the dust, but that their souls will go to be with Jesus in Paradise, a garden like the Garden of Eden, there to await the end of this present evil age.

Then, one day, Jesus will return. He will be clothed with the resurrection body in which he rose from the dead. Then, the followers of Jesus will also be re-clothed in resurrection bodies, citizens of the new world and of an Eternal City whose builder and maker is God.

The choice

But that is not the whole story. A different fate awaits those who refuse the offer of eternal life in Jesus Christ. People who prefer the life of this present world over the promise of the life of the world to come, who prefer to go on living life their own way instead of living it the way that God has planned, will inherit the inevitable consequences of their choices. They will lose what they have lived for in this world. They will experience remorse and regret, and in the end come only to that final destination that the Bible calls the Second Death.

Life after death

Many of us are unsure what form life after death takes. We do know that the Bible speaks of the dead in Christ being with Jesus. They still recognise one another and enjoy the company of those they love. The Bible also speaks of those who lament that they are separated from God the Father and from Jesus His Son, because they chose another way. But for everyone this is essentially a time of waiting until the final stage: the return of Jesus, the resurrection of the body, and the beginning of the new age and the new creation. Just as the body of Jesus was raised from the dead, but in a changed form, so, at the second coming of Jesus our earthly bodies will be raised from the dead, in a changed form. It is in these resurrection bodies that we shall live forever in the new world that God is preparing for those who love him.

For those who accept this hope that Jesus offers, there is a future of unimaginable and unending happiness in a new and perfect world, without all the troubles and tragedies of this present world – a world full of love, joy and peace. However, there is no way in which the teaching of Jesus, and the Bible in general, can be understood to offer such a future for all. There is always the call to repentance, a sense of crisis as we face death and the life of the world to come, the need for choice and decision about what we want, here and hereafter.

The Good News

The Good News is that we do not have to wait, even now there is a way out of the perplexities and dilemmas of this present world. There is the possibility of a new birth into a new life. The failures and shortcomings of our former lives are forgiven and left behind. Through the life, death and resurrection of Jesus, the way has been opened for us to have a future entirely different from our past, both here and now and in the world to come.

The importance of talking about life after death

What could be more important than the question of our eternal destiny? Is there such a thing at all? If so, is it good or bad? It is astonishing how little thought we seem to give to these questions, and how little they feature in our conversations.

It is important to talk about all this long before the approach of death itself. Indeed, the best place to sort it out as best we can is at the beginning of life, not at the end of it. The conclusions that we draw, and the faith by which we live, will make an immeasurable difference to the way in which we live our lives, as well as to the way in which we die.

It is difficult to say when the first intimations of mortality strike us; there is no rule. For some it may be in childhood.

My own experience was that when I was nine years old, lying in bed one night, I felt my heart beating and realised that one day my heart would stop and I would be dead. I panicked and pushed the thought away.

I did not talk about this to anyone at the time. Looking back, I should have talked to my father, a man of steadfast faith. For other people, the awful awareness of mortality may not strike them until later, but whenever it dawns on us that we are mortal, we need to talk about it with whoever might seem to be able to help. It is only by talking about it that some of our doubts and confusions about life after death will be clarified, some of our fears relieved, and some of our questions answered so that, whenever death actually comes, we can face it with as much faith and hope as mortals can expect to enjoy.

Sharing the Good News

It is also important for Christian believers to talk to their friends and families about life after death, both in order to share with them the good news of God's plan and of Jesus' offer of eternal life, but also in order to warn them of the consequences of rejecting this offer.

The things of this world are transient; the things of the world to come are eternal. What are 70 or 80 years in this world compared to eternity in the world to come? It is important that we live the whole of our earthly lives with an eternal perspective, starting when we are young, lest, in the search for and the enjoyment of this world's passing pleasures and achievements, we miss what is the most important thing of all: eternal life with God in his Kingdom.

Faith

Finally, in this life, we walk by faith and not by sight.

Here by way of encouragement are words from an old Christian hymn:

> My knowledge of that life is small,
> The eye of faith is dim;
> But 'tis enough that Christ knows all,
> And I shall be with him.

Richard Baxter

Questions to help us talk to others about life after death

How do you feel about dying?

What is the story of you and God?

Do you expect any experience of life after death?

Resources

The list of resources below will guide you to places where you can find out more about Jesus and about the new life that he came to bring. The best resource, however, is a local church, a local fellowship of believers who love Jesus and believe in the Bible, in which all this is revealed.

Concerning the life of Jesus:

The Bible: in particular, the Gospels of Matthew, Mark, Luke, and John.

Books about the evidence for resurrection of Jesus:

Morrison, Frank, *Who Moved the Stone?* (Authentic Media) – a classic.

Craig, William Lane, *The Son Rises* (Wipf and Stock, 2000)

Habermas, Gary *The Case for the Resurrection of Jesus* (Kregel Publications, 2004)

Books about the Christian hope:

Wright, Tom *Surprised by Hope* (SPCK, 2011)

Down, Martin *The Christian Hope: a Guide to Life after Death* (Rehoboth Media, 2016)

Bible texts from the New Testament specifically about the life of the world to come:

The hope of everlasting life:
John 3:16, John 5:24-30, John 6:35-40, John 10:27-29, John 11:25-27, 1 Corinthians 15:1-26

What happens when we die:
Luke 23:42-43, Luke 16:19-31, John 14:1-6

The choice:
Matthew 7:13-14, John 3:17-21

The return of Jesus:
Matthew 24:29-31, 1 Thessalonians 4:13-18

The Last Judgement:
Revelation 20:11-15

The New Creation:
1 Corinthians 15:35-57, 2 Corinthians 4:16 – 5:10,
Revelation 21:1 – 22:21.

10

FACING UP TO FEAR

Martin Down

Fear is something that is felt by every living creature. For animals, it is the natural reaction to a situation of imminent danger, stimulating whatever evasive action the animal can take. But for human beings, with the gift or curse of foresight, fear and anxiety also comes from the apprehension of some future danger, real or imagined. The threat may be of pain, loss, hardship, or of course, death. No one is immune from these fears; they are part of the human condition, common to us all. So how should we cope with fear and anxiety?

There are rational fears and irrational fears: rational fears are fears of some real hardship or suffering; irrational fears or phobias are fears that have no ground in reality, but are some dark figment of our imagination. A fear of spiders is not usually the fear of poisonous bites, but some irrational fear of spiders' legs. On the other hand, a fear of heights has a more rational basis, inasmuch as a fall from a great height is a real danger to life and limb. Fears of pain, sickness and death are rational fears; the fear of doctors and hospitals as such is irrational: all the staff in surgeries, clinics or wards are concerned only for our welfare.

In contemporary Western culture, there is such a powerful conviction that human life is all about health and happiness that it is not surprising that people seem to be afraid to talk about dying and death. These are usually regarded as negative and painful experiences that we are anxious to avoid. Moreover, there may be a lingering suspicion or fear that talking about these things may bring them nearer. In particular, there is a reluctance to talk about the possibility of dying to a sick person, lest the prospect depresses them or saps their will to fight against the illness that is threatening them. The will to live is after all an important factor in survival.

Fear of dying and fear of death are not the same thing. People often say, 'I am not afraid of death, but I am afraid of dying.' I am never sure that I believe them or, if I do, that they have their priorities right. By the fear of dying they mean the fear of the process of dying, the fear of the physical and mental pain involved in the progress of their final illness, and the consequences of leaving this world with regard to those left behind. As far as physical pain goes, today this is probably an exaggerated fear: pain-killing drugs that will be readily prescribed by the medical profession during our final illness are highly effective in relieving the worst of our pains.

Mental pain in the face of dying is a different and more intractable problem: the sense of powerlessness to control our lives, the prospect of separation from loved ones, both for us and for them, the frustration at hopes for the future being cut short, the anxiety over things left undone, all these, and perhaps the fear of the unknown after death, are fears that require a different sort of treatment.

Fear of what happens after I die is a very specific fear and a very rational one. Is death just the end of everything, or, perhaps more frightening, is there some form of life after death? Does the character of that life depend on what sort of a life I have lived here on earth? Will my darkest secrets be exposed? Is there some sort of reckoning, some sort of purgation or punishment to be endured? If so, what can I do about it? Is there anything I can do to prepare for such an eventuality? The prospect of death can bring us face-to-face with that sense of guilt that we all carry with us, because we have all fallen short of even our own standards of right and wrong, let alone God's. As the old Prayer Book of the Church of England says, 'We have left undone those things which we ought to have done, and we have done those things which we ought not to have done'.

We have looked at the questions that arise about life after death in the chapter above, and, in particular, what we can do from a Christian point of view to prepare for it: repent and believe in Jesus. There is no substitute for thinking through these issues and taking the necessary steps for ourselves, and the sooner in our lives we do it, the better. It is only too easy for us when life is going well and we are in rude health to postpone this task. But when the real possibility of dying arises, when death advances from over the horizon to the present, or the near future, we will wish that we had acquired some well-considered and settled faith, one way or another, to support us in our dying hours. It is not a good idea to put this enquiry off until we are on our death-beds, possibly in a state of drug-induced semi-consciousness. Do it now.

Whatever the fears that trouble us, there are some steps that we can take that will help us to bear, if not resolve, our uncertainties.

Talking about our fears

Whatever the nature of our fears the first step is to talk about them. Anxieties only grow and multiply when we try to ignore them or keep them in the dark. Bringing our fears into the light by talking to someone about them, often enables us to see them from a new perspective. If our confidant is a person of wisdom and experience we may find help and comfort in their counsel and advice. Even if all they can offer is their love and support, a hand to hold, this itself relieves the sense of being alone in our distress.

> Supporters of Liverpool Football Club apparently derived much strength after the Hillsborough disaster, and go on deriving strength from the assurance that by merely being supporters of the same team, 'they will never walk alone'.

Whatever the group to which we belong, the football supporters' club, our family, our friends, the church, our colleagues at work, if there are people within our circle with whom we can share our fears and anxieties, the sentiment of the Liverpool song is true enough: when we walk through the storms of life we draw strength from companions who will walk through it with us, whatever the outcome may be. So a first step in dealing with fears and anxiety is to seek out a trusted listener and 'open our grief'.

It may turn out that our fears are purely imaginary. The fears that disturb us in the dead of night are often revealed as no more than fantasies when we draw the curtains in the morning. Letting another sort of light into our nightmares as we reveal them to a friend can have the same wholesome effect. We can see how silly we have been to worry; how unlikely or unreal the dangers that we have imagined. Of course, not all our anxieties are groundless, but naming them and talking about them helps us to see reality for what it is, and that is the first step to coping with it. That is the first step to mastering our fears and dealing with the future: talking about it.

Phobias

True phobias are the most difficult to deal with. Confessing and talking about them can help. But so deep are the roots of these fears that we are not easily delivered from them. In a Christian context, prayer for deliverance in the name of Jesus can help in some instances, but in all cases there is usually a longer process of confronting and overcoming habitual reactions of fear. But even in the worst cases, having a companion and helper who will accompany us through our times of fear is a source of strength.

Doing something about it

'Thinking will not overcome fear but action will.'

W. Clement Stone, American self-help author

The second step in dealing with our fears and anxieties is to consider what action we can take to improve the situation. When we are anxious about the progress of our illness or the approach of death, we need to talk about it openly with our medical advisors, our family and friends. The sort of conversations that we ought to be having are outlined in this book. What are the options for treatment? What are the prospects of recovery or of deterioration in our condition? How can the medical profession help us to cope with whatever the future may hold?

If our days are limited, we must go on to ask how we can make the best use of the time left to us here on earth.

In the film *The Bucket List* two characters in the same hospital room find themselves facing the same terminal diagnosis. Carter is a blue-collar mechanic; Edward Cole is a billionaire businessman. Carter has drawn up a 'bucket list' of the things he wants to do before he dies, and Cole offers to finance a last trip round the world for them both to fulfil their dreams. They go sky-diving; they visit the Taj Mahal and the Pyramids. But by the end of the film they have both discovered that the most important thing in life is love, and both in different ways have returned to and been reconciled with their families.

This is a good guide for anyone facing such a prospect: the best use to which we can put the rest of our lives, however long or short they may be, is to invest our time and energy in bringing happiness to others, especially those nearest and dearest to us.

Perhaps the most important task in this area of personal relationships is to make peace, before it is too late, with anyone whom we have quarrelled with or whom we are aware of having hurt. A letter or a phone call, with a word of apology or regret, may have been long owing. On the other hand, it may be a word of forgiveness that we need to speak. We may need to make some more tangible reparation or amends for things that we have done wrong. Such efforts may or may not succeed in mending a relationship: just as it takes two to make a quarrel, so it takes two to make it up. But if we have made a gesture in the right direction, we shall at least die knowing that we have done our best, and however our overtures have been received, we shall be able to die in peace. The most important relationship of all that we need to put right is our relationship with God.

These activities, whether fulfilling our ambitions or attending to our personal relationships before it is too late, are activities that are constructive and helpful, but there is a frenetic sort of activity that is merely escapist and unhelpful. As a way of escaping our fears, this sort of activity is futile and counter-productive. This is because our fears will not be banished by it but will lie in wait for us, springing up again in the slow watches of the night, or catching us unawares in some unguarded moment in the day time. Fears have to be faced and confronted, not avoided and buried.

'Fear not'

In the end, I know no real remedy for fear of any sort other than faith. Friends can give us false assurances that 'things will turn out alright'. But things do not always turn out alright. We do suffer illness and infirmity; we do suffer pain and loss. One day, if not now then later, we will all have to die. There is no escaping these realities, though our present, materialistic, Western culture is not in touch with them and does not want to recognise them. That is why they cause us so much anxiety when they do draw near. It is God alone who can both say to us, 'Fear not', and give us good reason not to fear.

Here are some of the great 'fear nots' from the prophecy of Isaiah: 'fear nots' that can speak to our hearts at any time but especially in times of sickness and weakness.

'Fear not, for I am with you; be not dismayed for I am your God.' (Isaiah 41:10)

'I, the Lord your God, hold your right hand; it is I who say to you, "Fear not, I will help you".' (Isaiah 41:13)

'Fear not, for I have redeemed you.' (Isaiah 43:1)

We, the authors of this book, all believe that it is Jesus alone (as God in human form) who can set us free from our guilt and fears. By his death and resurrection, he has paid the price for our sins and overcome the power of the grave. In the night in which he was betrayed, he looked suffering and death full in the face and spoke to his disciples about these things, both for himself and for them. That evening, he spoke to them for a long time, over supper and on the way to the Garden of Gethsemane, beginning and finishing with these words:

'Do not let your hearts be troubled. Trust in God; trust also in me....'

'I have told you these things, so that in me you may have peace. In this world you will have trouble. But take heart! I have overcome the world.' (John 14:1 and 16:33)

Jesus himself shrank from the pain and suffering that would be involved in his death. In the Garden of Gethsemane, he prayed to God that he might be spared. But there was no other way for him to take away the sin that separates us from God. The disciples were confused and dismayed at the prospect of his death and, like all of us, afraid of suffering and death for themselves. They shared with us the same natural shrinking from these calamities, from which, in one form or another, there is no escape. Jesus said, 'In this world you will have trouble.' Notice the realism here; Jesus was not giving them any false assurances. They had to face these things, and so do we. But with him we can face them with peace and confidence, rather than with anxiety and fear.

Trust in God and trust in Jesus, who has trodden the path before us, is the key to walking through the valley of the shadow of death without fear. The apostle John, towards the end of his life, wrote, 'Perfect love drives out fear.' (1 John 4:18) Few of us can claim that we have achieved such perfect love that we have no fear at all, or have such perfect knowledge of the love of God for us, that we have no fear at all – though that is how it should be. But as we grow up in faith, so we grow out of fear.

The Good Shepherd promises that he will be with us as we walk through the valley of the shadow of death (Psalm 23:4). Who knows, until we reach that place, what that actually means?

When my own father, a man of strong and lifelong faith, was dying, our family was gathered round his bed. We prayed and sang hymns over him quietly as he lay peacefully with his eyes shut, either unconscious or asleep. The nurse came and turned him over in the bed, and in his last moments, he was lying on his side facing the wall beside which sat my mother and I. My father's breaths became shallower and shallower and less and less frequent. At length, without any warning, he opened his eyes wide and looked straight through my mother and me and straight through the wall behind us. It seemed as if he saw and greeted someone coming to fetch him. We all held our breath for about half a minute. Then he closed his eyes, breathed his last, and died.

Who knows what he saw? But I like to think that he saw Jesus fulfilling his word, 'I will come back and take you to be with me, that you also may be where I am' (John 14:3). I pray that it will be like that for me – and for you. Trust in God the Father and in Jesus the Son of God.

Questions to help us talk to people about their fears
Are you afraid?
What can be done to help you?

11

PRAYING FOR HEALING

Gareth Tuckwell

Here are two stories about prayer for healing within one family.

Prayer for healing – a son

'It is four in the morning. The crying of our six month old goes on and on ... and on. I can picture his determined red face as the crying reached that "I'm never going to stop" intensity that demands attention. I carry him downstairs – the Christmas tree lights showing the way ... then I find my balance thrown by an unseen pile of books ... a cry, then quietness. Paul and I arrived at the foot of the stairs; I am shaken and bruised but he is strangely still.

'Having just set up a prayer chain across our church, I stumble out an account of the accident and Paul's need for healing. Soon hundreds are praying for him across churches and countries. Vomiting, drowsy, blue lights; then paralysis, a limp right side. CAT scan; two-thirds of his skull is filled with blood. "Maybe a 30% chance of survival" – three hours of neurosurgery accompanied by parental numbness and prayer with anointing for healing on the ward. Anxious days of waiting.

'Now Paul is 30 with a good degree, a job he loves, and a strong Christian faith. He is a keen tennis player, a caring and discerning young man with a prominent scar usually hidden by hair: my scar remains inside. Thank you, Father God, for the power of prayer, for your amazing healing and for the skill of the surgeon who was there for us.'

Prayer for healing – a father

'Another year, another Christmas: my father is dying, struggling to stay in control in the face of confusion from overwhelming infection, despite ongoing prayer for his physical healing. He had taken Communion a few days before, and at the time he said to his vicar that his healing had taken place and that a depression that had overwhelmed him during this illness had lifted. "I am now ready for that great adventure after death that I have always believed in," he declared. I sit at his bedside and take his hand. My audible prayer is now not for physical healing but for the man I love to be spared indignity and further suffering; (for him, loss of control would be as painful as an open wound). A hot hand squeezes mine as if in agreement – as if my cry to God is echoing around the jangling neurones of his mind.

'What might have lasted hours or days is over; my father looks refreshed, peaceful and asleep. I pay my last respects and help the district nurse to give him a last "wash and brush up", before tidying the bed.

'At this moment, all the reality of life seems present – illness, death, humanity and eternal life. No more struggle. My father looks at home and secure – there is a sense that he has made it and all is well. The stillness of the room is deafening. It reminds me of the hush of excitement and exhaustion that surrounds mother and child when labour is over and a new life has begun. Somehow appropriate to Christmas and to death, so the Christian believes.'

By the time we reach middle age, most of us have cried out to God in times of life-threatening crisis, whatever our belief. For Christians there is an added dilemma. The Bible shows time and again how Jesus healed those who came to him. The Bible gives Christians a clear instruction to continue His mission and ministry, and many pray for sick people, confident that Jesus heals today. Sometimes there is remarkable recovery or a miraculous one. But often the illness takes its relentless course.

What is healing?
Our model of health is shaped by our fear of death, so that cure of disease naturally becomes a supreme value. Resources for the prolongation of life, such as fourth-line chemotherapies for treating widespread cancer, become a headline concern, one that the tabloid press loves to pick up and run with. Our understanding of health and healing must not be captive to the fear of death, but nor must it deny it.

Perhaps health and healing are found in relationship: to God himself, to ourselves (in accepting responsibility for who we are, rather than looking in the mirror and longing to be different), to our community (our neighbours both locally and further afield) and lastly in relationship to the environment as stewards of our God-given resources. Perhaps healing is to be in body, mind, spirit, emotions and relationships as we believe God intends for us – a journey we are all on until we reach the gates of Heaven. Healing brings wellbeing and a sense of coherence. We are restored with the possibility of fulfilling the purpose for which we were created.

I have found that Moltmann's picture of true health can be incredibly helpful at the bedside, especially in palliative care when a friend is facing their mortality and we are wondering just how to pray: 'Our society defines health as the capacity for work and a capacity for enjoyment, but true health is something quite different. True health is the strength to live, the strength to suffer, the strength to die. Health is not a condition of my body; it is the power of my soul to cope with the varying conditions of my body.'[1]

So what does the Christian expect when he or she claims that Jesus heals today? We know that our bodies are remarkable at recovery. A cut finger or a broken bone will usually heal, sometimes despite the treatment! We see how healthcare professionals are key players in treatment and care; many Christians would see them as used by God, just as medication and medical advances are brought about by the intellect God has given us. We also know that death is inevitable, and the timing of that is often beyond the control of man. In Europe, widespread loss of Christian belief, partly due to the advance of scientific discovery and the distraction of materialism, has resulted in a fear of death which has drained the word 'health' of its truly human dimension.

How should we pray?

So perhaps prayer for healing should not be focussed so much on the performing of physical miracles but rather more on seeing the healing power and presence of Jesus transforming lives? How then should we be praying for healing? When we pray for someone we love who is sick, do we expect God to answer? Do we really listen to God for that person? Do we wonder why God seems to heal some and not others, in terms of physical cure?

'This, then, is how you should pray: Our Father in heaven, hallowed be your name, your kingdom come, your will be done on earth as it is in heaven...' (Jesus' teaching on prayer in Luke 11:2-4).

A different healing

Cathy arrived at Burrswood Hospital one Saturday when I was the admitting doctor on duty. She arrived by ambulance, in a wheelchair, looking sullen, pale and withdrawn. There were three admissions and my son's birthday party to get to, so inside I felt hurried. Cathy was 32 and some months ago she had jumped off the balcony of her home after having a row with her drunken husband. She had broken her spine and was paralysed from the waist down. Her Christian faith was not quite extinguished by the desolation of her situation. 'What are you hoping for?' I asked.

She put her hands on her paralysed legs and said, 'I just want to walk again and tell people about Jesus.' My hurried mind wondered how to pray. Being a doctor makes prayers for miracles more difficult, even when I have seen them. Then the Lord's Prayer came to me. 'Lord Jesus, together we pray for your Kingdom to come in Cathy's life and for her to be open to receive all you have for her at this time.' Cathy did receive ... she left her sense of guilt and failure at the foot of the Cross, she had physiotherapy, hydrotherapy, prayer with the laying on of hands and anointing. When she left for home ten days later everyone said how different she looked. Cathy was radiant, but her legs were still paralysed.

Time went by and, four years later, I was standing in the main entrance to the hospital, when Cathy turned up, still in her wheelchair. 'I'm so happy. I trained as a Lay Pastoral Assistant and now I go around the town sharing God's love and truth with those I meet. I'm healed ... no, really I am!' she said as she pulled her leaden legs into a better position.

Why don't we always get the answer we want when we pray? Christian faith is not always problem-solving; more often it is mystery-encountering. As some have discovered in their progressive disease and pain: 'The trust one has to develop in God lies far deeper, in the knowledge that he will be present in the deepest waters, in the most acute pain and, in some appreciation of his will to transform things. No cheap belief in him as insurance will serve.' (Professor Margaret Spufford, 1989, on her own experience of a lifetime of illness and that of her daughter, who died aged 22.)[2]

Those of us who are Christians have to get away from believing that healing inevitably follows faith, that healing must always mean cure. If we believe in the resurrection, why do we see death as a disaster? Why do some people have an endless desire to see miracles day by day, rather than to see and know God in the nitty gritty of everyday life? Is it because we live in an instant age where there are seemingly answers to everything and if God is greater and God is love, then surely he will answer the shopping list of needs that are our heart cry! And yet we then discover how false optimism can destroy hope. Maybe magic is asking God to do our will whilst prayer is asking God to work in and through us, by *His* power, to do *His* will. We have to seek the mind of Christ, to hold our pastoral hearts and professional minds alongside the certainty that Jesus heals today. We need to see healing, above all, in the context of the prayer that Jesus taught us, that His Kingdom might come in the lives of those for whom we pray.

The late Bishop Morris Maddocks, adviser to the Archbishops on the ministry of health and healing (1983-1995), was inspired when, in a television interview, he redefined Christian healing and took the wind out of the sails of the interviewer who was trying to pour scorn on the miraculous: 'Christian healing,' said Morris, 'is Jesus Christ meeting you at the point of your need.'[3]

Can prayer for physical healing be unhelpful?
Hospice staff not uncommonly have to manage contrasting needs. Their patient with advanced progressive disease has

just come to terms with the fact that death is not far distant, when a group of Christian friends turn up asking permission to pray at this person's bedside and claim the healing they believe Jesus will bring. It is wise to ask the group who are praying expectantly and fervently for a return to physical health to pray in the chapel or prayer room, whatever is provided. Walls are no barrier to prayer but even prayer in the name of Jesus and prayed in love can disrupt the peaceful letting-go of a dying person. It is so hard to let go of the one we love and have cared for, and even harder to give them permission to let go of this life so they feel set free to move on to the fullness of life eternal, without any sense of having lost the battle for life on earth.

How should we pray?

Andy Drain, a young 'just become' cardiothoracic surgeon who was dying of leukaemia wrote in his stunning book, *Code Red*:[4] 'So rather than pray for the weight to be lifted from our shoulders, sometimes we should just pray for stronger shoulders.' He was confident of God's hand on his dying and had let go of the need to ask 'why?'

'I hope we will move forward to a day when death will not be regarded as a sordid end but rather as an act of dignity on the part of someone dying well. An act worthy of a person made in the image of God: an act which, it is true, ends one phase of their personhood but which ushers in a new phase for which indeed they were created, that phase when, for the Christian believer, the vision of God dimly seen here, is fulfilled in the bliss of life eternal.' (Lord Coggan, former Archbishop of Canterbury).

Perhaps a God who heals some and not others is unacceptable to so many because it leaves us not in control. And yet, when we become like a little child who doesn't understand everything but still trusts, then the way forward is incredibly simple. God holds all the reins and we come along for the ride, just as Cathy did!

Just as Jesus read from the prophet Isaiah's writings in the synagogue in Nazareth and outlined his work on earth at that time, so we are called to take up the mantle today: God has chosen you and me and sent us to bring good news to the poor, to heal the broken-hearted, to announce release to captives and freedom to those in prison. God has sent you and me to proclaim that the time has come when He will save His people.[5]

I conclude with a Franciscan benediction:

May God bless us with discomfort at easy answers, half-truths, and superficial relationships, so that we may live true to our hearts;

May God bless us with disquiet at compromise, prescriptive solutions, and political expediency, so that we may work with compassion for a better way, for freedom, healing and peace;

May God bless us with tears, so that we may be set free to reach out our hands to bring comfort, and our hearts, that we may share in the pain and joy of those who are vulnerable, sick and marginalised;

Finally, may God bless us with enough 'foolishness' to believe that prayer in the name of Jesus can make a difference in our world, so that, in His name, we can do what others claim cannot be done. Particularly, as we seek to bring the all-surpassing love of Jesus into our communities, as we look to Him to bring health and healing ... and one day, a good death, to all those who cross our path, including those clinging to the bottom rung.

Amen

Questions to help us talk to others about healing

• What are you hoping for now?

• What do you want God to do for you?

Notes

[1] Jürgen Moltmann: *God in Creation*, Fortress Publishing, 1993.

[2] Spufford, Margaret, *Celebration* (Continuum International Publishing, 1996)

[3] The Right Reverend Morris Maddocks, who died on January 19, 2008, aged 79, was Suffragan Bishop of Selby from 1972 to 1983, then adviser to the Archbishops of Canterbury and York on the ministry of health and healing. This change of role, which involved much more than the offering of advice, was driven by a deep conviction that health of body, mind and spirit were closely related and too important to be left solely to doctors or to charismatic 'healers'. He regarded collaboration between the healing professions as essential and believed that concern for health should be a normal part of the work of every local church.

[4] Andrew J Drain, *Code Red* (Christian Medical Fellowship, 2010)

[5] See Luke 4:19 and Isaiah 61:1.

12

PRACTICAL MATTERS

Martin Down

In preparing this chapter, I have drawn on the professional expertise of a solicitor, David Wright, and a funeral director, Paul Littleproud, for whose help and advice I am extremely grateful. I have also drawn on my own experience as a clergyman of the Church of England for many years, and as the older child of two parents, who are both now deceased.

At the time of death

You may have some say about where you choose to die. In the case of a death that is foreseen, you may be able to decide whether you want to die in hospital, in a nursing home or at home. It will depend on the nature of your illness and the requirements of treating or caring for you. Most people will say that they would rather die at home. Sometimes this is possible with the help of visiting carers or nurses to supplement the care of family members. In other cases, it may be necessary for us to be in hospital or residential care. For some of us, this will not be a choice that we have the chance to make. A sudden death, at home, in the street or even abroad, means that someone else will have to cope with the consequences for us.

If you die in hospital or residential care then the process of confirming your death and certifying its cause will usually be straightforward. If on the other hand you die at home, someone with you or finding you will have to summon help as soon as possible. Depending on the time of day, they should telephone your doctor or dial 111, for someone to attend. If, of course, there is any doubt about your state, living or dead, then someone should immediately telephone 999 for an ambulance.

If a doctor or paramedic attending the home certifies that you have indeed died, then there is no need for an ambulance to be called. Your body can be taken straight to a Chapel of Rest by an undertaker, and prepared there for your funeral. In times gone by, people would commonly be washed, laid out and prepared for burial by a neighbour or a friend, and kept in the house until the funeral could take place. But such a practice is rare today and the job is usually entrusted to a professional funeral director.

If you have the misfortune to die in some public place or abroad then there is no alternative but for someone to call for an ambulance and let the medical services take over.

Obtaining a Medical Certificate

Death creates a good deal of work and expense for those who are left behind. Immediately, they will have to go through various legal formalities to do with obtaining a doctor's Medical Certificate which records the cause of death. The process of obtaining such a Medical Certificate will be more or less easy for our relatives, depending on whether we died in hospital, under the recent care of a General Practitioner, or neither, as in the case of a sudden or unexpected death. In the last case, reference will have to be made to the Coroner and there may have to be a *post mortem* and an inquest. This may delay any funeral by several days or even weeks. Meanwhile, the body will have to be kept in a mortuary or chapel of rest. It may be a good idea to contact a funeral director immediately, without waiting for the issue of a Medical Certificate. It can sometimes take several days to obtain this Certificate and meanwhile provisional funeral arrangements can be put in hand.

Registering a death

Once a Medical Certificate has been issued, it must be taken to the local Registrar. Contact details for the Registrar's Office can normally be found in the telephone directory or online. It is a good idea to telephone the Office to arrange an appointment for registering the death rather than simply turning up and having to wait a long time. If you are registering the death of a close relative or friend, this can be a very emotional, even painful occasion so it is wise to ask someone you know to accompany you.

The Registrar will register the death and furnish copies of the entry in the Register for the purposes of winding up our affairs. A copy of this entry – which is customarily called the 'Death Certificate' – will be given to the person notifying the death. It is possible, and usually sensible, to obtain, for a small fee, further copies which may need to be shown as evidence of the death to banks and pension funds and similar organisations, some of whom do not accept photocopies but insist on an original certificate. There is also a scheme by which the Registrar can arrange for you to 'Tell us once': this enables the Registrar to notify all the necessary government agencies on behalf of the person registering that you have died. This will save a great deal of work. The Registrar will also issue a 'green form', authorising Burial or Cremation. With this in hand our next of kin can begin to make or confirm arrangements for a funeral with the undertaker or funeral director.

Finding a Will

As soon as possible after our death, someone needs to find the Will and start to act in accordance with its provisions. These may include instructions or wishes with regard to the funeral, as well as longer term arrangements about the disposal of our property. If there is no Will, then someone, usually a relative or solicitor, will have to begin the process of applying to the Probate Registry for a grant of Letters of Administration in a case of intestacy. When it comes to the disposal of our property, the services of a solicitor are essential whether we left a Will or not, in order to make sure that what is done is in accordance with the law and is beyond legal challenge, either immediately or in the future.

There are various people who will guide those who are left behind through these various stages of settling our affairs – the doctor, the Registrar, the funeral director, and the solicitor – but the whole process will be easier and smoother if some of the issues have been discussed while we are still alive. Our wishes and thoughts about these things are important and should be made known, which is another reason why we should talk about dying before it is too late.

Lasting Power of Attorney

Our first conversations or thoughts about putting our own affairs in order should be around the drawing up of a Lasting Power of Attorney and the making of a Will. It is sensible for anyone who has acquired either a family or some real estate to do both, however young they may be, and however far off their death may seem. Most of us have financial responsibilities with regard both to our property and to those dependent on us. During our lives we attend to these things ourselves, but there will come a time when we can no longer do so, either through the deterioration of our physical or mental capacities or through death. We need to recognise that such a deterioration or death may occur gradually over a longer or shorter period of time, or come suddenly, like a thief in the night, and therefore make sure that we act before it is too late.

So long as we are able, we decide what to spend, what to save, what to give away, and to whom. We fill in our tax returns, pay our bills, and manage our own bank accounts. If there comes a time before we die when through incapacity we cannot do these things, someone else will have to do them for us. The way to make provision for this is through a Lasting Power of Attorney (LPA). To find out how to do this, go to www.gov.uk/power-of-attorney/overview or ask a solicitor or enquire at your local Citizen's Advice Bureau. By signing such a document, we authorise someone we trust to deal with our affairs in a way that is in our best interests, and hopefully in the way in which we would wish them to be dealt with, had we still been able to do so. The person we choose to do this may be a relative, perhaps a spouse, or a friend, or it may be a trusted professional such as a solicitor or accountant. But it is important not to wait before doing this, especially as we grow older, in case some medical or physical accident occurs out of the blue, depriving us of the ability to create such a Power.

Making a Will

The way we order our affairs after death is by way of a Will. If a person has left no Will, it is called an intestacy.

Some years ago, a lady in her eighties died; she was a single lady with only distant relatives who had never been involved in her life. She owned her own house and had a substantial estate. A member of her church, who was a retired solicitor, was asked to make a search for the Will. On gaining access to the house, it soon became clear that the lady had been an inveterate hoarder; every room in her house was covered in the accumulated detritus of the last years of her life. It took many days of searching before the conclusion was reached that she had never made a Will: she had died intestate. The result was that the estate passed, not to the friends who had cared for her and had been close to her for many years, nor to the church or a charity that she might have wished to support, but to those distant relatives, some of whom had never even known of her existence.

A Will can only be made by someone who has the mental capacity to do so. This is another reason for thinking, talking and doing something about it before it is too late. The services of a solicitor are invaluable if we want to be sure that the Will is drawn up in the proper form, properly signed and witnessed, and phrased so as to avoid legal ambiguity. There are many complications about making a Will, for example, leaving property to an underage person such as a grandchild and making arrangements for the legacy to be properly managed until that child comes of age, or taking steps to minimise Inheritance Tax in a way that is honourable and legal. Minor alterations can be made to a Will later by signing a Codicil, but this must be signed in the same way as the Will itself. A Will can always be revoked by destruction, or by making a new Will. But it is always wise to seek the advice of a solicitor. Again, the telephone directory, Yellow Pages, a local directory of business or the internet, will supply a list of suitably qualified practitioners, but a word with friends may be useful in identifying a solicitor who is friendly, efficient and affordable.

In recent years, and in the light of modern medical advances, some people now also consider making what is known as a Living Will or an Advance Directive, which is a document specifying the treatments that we may or may not wish to undergo in the case of a terminal illness. We have treated this subject at greater length in chapter 3: *Difficult*

Decisions and Appendix 3.

Many of these issues could and should be addressed long before the end comes. It does not in any way hasten the day of our death to make a Will and to talk to our loved ones about what we want to put into it. A discussion with a husband or wife is the least we can offer to someone who has spent the best years of their life with us. A family discussion involving children and even grandchildren can also prepare the way for a division of our property that will satisfy those we leave behind and not lead to quarrels and jealousy.

One last thought: it is no good making a Will or a Lasting Power of Attorney if they cannot be found when they are required. If they are held on our behalf by a solicitor, the name and address of the solicitor should be made known. If we keep such documents at home, let us put them in a safe place and then tell at least one trusted person exactly where they are to be found; not just in a particular room, but indicating whereabouts in the room they are kept. My father, unlike the old lady whose story you have just read, left all his papers in a drawer in his bureau, and told me where to find them, before he died.

Planning a funeral

The first question that has to be decided is whether we want to be buried or cremated. The Roman Catholic Church once forbade cremation, but has since changed its teaching and now permits it. Beyond that, in a Christian or secular culture, it is a matter of individual or family preference. Some people prefer the idea of a grave in which their bones are laid to rest and over which can stand a suitable memorial. Some especially like the idea of burial in a churchyard, though this is increasingly difficult as churchyards fill up. But in making such plans for burials and memorials, beware! There are usually strict rules both in churchyards and municipal cemeteries about what may and may not be done to mark a grave or commemorate the departed. It is wise to check with the relevant authorities before making firm plans. From the point of view of those who are left, some families like to have a grave to visit and perhaps to tend. For others this would be an unwelcome responsibility. For some a known and visible grave helps them to recognise the finality of death. But for others it works the other way and hinders them from letting go of the dead. In any case, in a heavily populated country where there are so many pressures on land use, many people appreciate the practicality of cremation.

There still remains the question of how to dispose of our ashes. There is no legal reason why they cannot be kept in a jar on the mantelpiece or in a box at the bottom of the wardrobe, but most people would prefer to have their ashes either scattered in a favourite spot, or interred in a cemetery or churchyard. There will be considerable costs involved in either burial or cremation, and the relative costs may be a factor in the decision that we, and our next of kin, finally make. As with the business of making a Will, it is often useful to discuss these options with a professional, in this case with a funeral director or undertaker, even before we have died.

Whatever our wishes, the costs of a funeral can be considerable. The most basic funeral now costs in the region of £3,000. This does not include the cost of the funeral wake or party for the mourners after the ceremony, nor the cost of any sort of memorial. A number of organisations offer pre-paid Funeral Plans. It is well to research the different options on the market. Beware especially of plans that tie you into using a particular firm of local undertakers. You may move before you die, or die away from home, in which case it may be expensive or inconvenient to use the services of the funeral director with whom you have taken out the pre-paid plan. On the other hand, there are other organisations that arrange pre-paid funeral plans which can be taken up with a network of undertakers all over the country from which you can choose at any time.

The funeral service

There will be many decisions to be made about the funeral when the time comes, some of which we may wish to make ourselves, rather than leave them solely to those who we leave behind. Cremation needs to be discussed as mentioned above. Religious services vary according to the faith community concerned, as we consider in the section below. A secular service or ceremony is certainly possible, and if we have spent our lives without entering a church or chapel then it is probably more honest to die in the same way. On the other hand, for an observant and faithful member of a Christian church or of any other religion, a funeral according to the rites and ceremonies of that faith is entirely appropriate and a comfort to those who mourn.

A Christian service will involve a choice of hymns or songs or other music, perhaps also of readings and prayers. Not only the undertaker, but also the Christian priest or minister, should be consulted about the appropriateness and practicality of such requests. The practice of reading passages of prose or poetry, or playing particular pieces of music associated with the deceased person, has become quite fashionable. Whether these are appropriate in the context of a faith-based service in which the focus is on God and the hope he has set before us, needs to be discussed with all those involved, and particularly the priest or minister. We ourselves may want to contribute to these choices before we die, and these are things about which it is helpful to have had conversations with those who will be responsible for carrying them out.

A secular funeral usually consists of a number of friends and relations paying tribute to our qualities in life, and reading passages of poetry or prose that meant something important to us or to them. Likewise, pieces of music may be played that in some way recall our lives or had special associations for us.

Other funeral arrangements

There will be many more practical questions that the undertaker will need to resolve with our relatives, many of which may never have occurred to us in life. The business of going to our final rest, like everything else in 21st-century Western life, is now heavily commercialised. We can depart not only in a black motor-car, but alternatively in a horse-drawn hearse, or on a motorbike and side-car, or even in a VW camper van. We can have a plain wooden coffin, or a psychedelic one, or a straw basket. Perhaps more mundanely, we can be dressed in a plain shroud or gown, or in clothes of our own choice. We may want to decide what we want the mourners to do about flowers or donations in our memory, what notices we want to be put in the press, what sort of a memorial, if any, we want: a stone in a cemetery or churchyard, an entry in a Book of Remembrance, a tree planted or a seat dedicated. We may be entirely indifferent to some or all of these matters, or we may have very clear ideas about them. Either way, we should make these wishes known before it is too late.

Other religious communities

For those who belong to Jewish, Muslim, Hindu, Buddhist or other Asian communities, there are often specific requirements about the treatment and disposal of the dead. For example, for Muslims, who form the largest non-

Christian religious community in Britain, cremation is 'haram': forbidden. For Muslims it is imperative to arrange the burial as quickly as possible after death. This involves clearing all financial matters for the deceased (such as debts), arranging a ritual bath, and wrapping the body in simple white cloths to symbolise the leaving behind of all earthly possessions. *Post mortem* examination to establish the cause of death represents for Muslims a desecration of the body, and, since it can rarely be performed immediately, it also represents an unwelcome delay of the burial, but may in some cases be a legal necessity.

Other religious communities, including Muslims and Jews, often have their own funeral directors, people who are familiar with their own religious or ethnic customs and can advise and arrange appropriate obsequies. Even within these communities there are those who are more or less observant of the traditional ceremonies, and they too need to discuss their wishes with those who going to be left behind, before it is too late.

'Before it is too late.'

This is a phrase that has occurred many times in this chapter, and it sums up the burden of it. There are many things that we ought to do in preparation for our own death while we still have the power and capacity to do them: making a Will and a Lasting Power of Attorney; thinking and talking about our funeral.

Ruth had spent her life as a pastoral counsellor, a calling for which she had a special gifting. In her fifties she had developed cancer. At first, therapy had seemed to be successful. But after some eight years the cancer returned and her consultant advised that she had only a few months to live. In fact she lived another two years, in which time she and her husband Andrew, himself a hospital consultant, spoke often of what lay ahead. Both were committed Christians and while they grieved at the idea of being parted they faced the future with a firm trust in God and in being reunited in the world to come. As for her funeral, Ruth had very clear ideas about where and how she wanted to be buried: she wanted to be buried in the country churchyard in which many of Andrew's family already rested, and where Andrew could be buried beside her when the time came. A visit to the parish and a conversation with the vicar revealed that this would be possible and so plans were made.

As the end drew near, Ruth and Andrew talked together about the funeral, discussed the hymns and the order of service. Ruth wanted some of her previous clients to be invited as well as family and friends. As someone who had counselled them in life she wanted to help them to let go of her in death, and to rely instead on God who is an ever-present help in trouble. She had helped them to live well and now she wanted to help them to die well. Ruth also wanted her funeral to include a celebration of Holy Communion, an unusual though not unheard of part of the last rites in the Church of England. Ruth herself believed that the service of Holy Communion was the most effective means of healing, both physical and emotional, available to Christians because of the intimate connection that it brings to Jesus the Healer, and indeed to the great company of those who rest in him.

Andrew and Ruth invited the funeral director whom they had chosen, to visit them in the days before Ruth died in order to make the necessary arrangements with him. This man confessed that only on a handful of occasions in a lifetime as an undertaker had he been invited to discuss a funeral with the person he was about to bury. But he remarked that he considered that it was extremely helpful, to him, to the person approaching death, and to the next of kin, to have had such a discussion, and he wished that more people would take such forethought and have the courage to talk about their death while they can.

In this book we have been encouraging people to talk about dying, and not least is this important in the context of putting our affairs in order, while we still have time. Below are some of the practical questions that we need to ask ourselves and possibly to ask other people near to us, especially as we and they grow older.

- Have you made a Will?
- Do you know what a Lasting Power of Attorney is?
- Have you thought about what sort of a funeral you want?

In my own experience it is not a morbid or depressing exercise to take the practical steps that will make life easier for those we leave behind whenever the time comes. On the contrary, it sets me free to enjoy the rest of my life, knowing that I have done all I can to smooth the way for those who will have to deal with my death whenever that comes. Be it sooner or later, I am free to go.

Resources

Citizens Advice Bureau can offer help and advice with any of these matters, either via their website,

https://www.citizensadvice.org.uk/relationships/death-and-wills/

or on the telephone 03 444 111 444 or in person at your local Citizens Advice Bureau.

There are many websites where information and advice can be found about putting your affairs in order before you die, for example:

Making a Will: www.gov.uk/make-will/overview

www.lawsociety.org.uk/for-the-public/common-legal-issues/making-a-will

Lasting Power of Attorney:

www.gov.uk/power-of-attorney/overview

What to do when someone dies:

www.gov.uk/after-a-death/overview

Arranging a funeral:

www.gov.uk/after-a-death/arrange-the-funeral

www.nafd.org.uk/funeral-advice/find-a-member

www.saif.org.uk/members-search

13

HOW WE CAN HELP

Philip Giddings and Elaine Sugden

As we said at the end of our first chapter, serious illness, dying and death itself pose profound questions which strike at the heart of what life is and our sense of identity. Whilst we do not pretend to have provided all the answers in this book, we are convinced that by encouraging people to *talk about dying* more openly we are offering a powerful way of helping one another as and when we have to face up to the questions and challenges which dying and death bring.

In this book we have used information gathered in our professional and general lives. Between us we have had many and varied experiences of family and friends who have died: those at the end of a long life, although sometimes only after lengthy suffering for them and others, as well as those who have died before birth, in infancy, young or mature adulthood. Some deaths have been sudden, others prolonged.

When we encounter the deep pain and emptiness of the loss of a loved one, particularly a spouse or a child, it is comforting to know not only that we are not unique in feeling as we do but also to see how others have navigated these paths before. Others too have felt, on top of their deeply bruised emotions, confused and overwhelmed by medical terms and administrative procedures. So we hope that we have helped in this book to explain and de-mystify the processes and procedures and to point to some resources which will be helpful in these painful situations.

We all need to think about our own death and any preparation we can make for it.

Whilst there is no adequate preparation for the severity of the emotional shock of losing a loved one, there is much that we can do by way of preparation to help ourselves, and those who will have the responsibility of caring for us when we are dying.

We started this book because few people talked about death but, as we have been writing, there has been increasing discussion. Several changes in society have provoked conversations in the media: the survival of the majority into a frail old age, with need of care from family, friends, medical staff and care homes; the assisted suicide debate; the rising incidence of bypassing a funeral with the body going straight to the crematorium for disposal, and not least the current cultural norm that patients should be given information about their diagnosis and treatment and that: 'any decisions about me should not be made without me'.[1]

'Too many people we love had not died in the way they would choose. Too many survivors were left feeling depressed, guilty, uncertain whether they'd done the right thing.'

'The difference between a good death and a hard death often seemed to hinge essentially on whether someone's wishes were expressed and respected. Whether they'd had a conversation about how they wanted to live toward the end.'

Ellen Goodman (*New York Times*)[2]

One way the death conversation has been explored is in 'Death Cafes'.[3] These occasional events have been held in several locations in the UK and are open to all. At a Death Cafe people drink tea, eat cake and discuss death. The stated aim 'is to increase awareness of death to help people make the most of their (finite) lives'.

A participant in a Death Cafe (2015) wrote: 'What we did all share were our own individual experiences of people, including oneself, who have gone through, or expect to go through the business of supporting people who are dying, by helping them to talk about the things that most concern them, which are common to people of strong, little, or no religious faith. It was valuable just to be able to talk with other people *objectively* about their several experiences of dealing with death, the importance of making a Will, of "resuscitation issues", of expressing their wishes about their funeral arrangements, ways of meeting the costs, and not least having the chance to listen to those whose approach to the subject differs significantly from one's own.'

The Church of England is running a project on the same lines called *Grave Talk*.[4] Tea and cake are also involved as participants discuss a range of questions about death: its meaning, practical issues, bereavement, funerals, etc.

'Churches are well-placed to host open conversations for people to explore the deeper questions of life and death.'

Revd David Primrose,
Director of Transforming Communities for Lichfield Diocese

A group of friends could decide to do something similar in a coffee morning or after a dinner meeting. We are not sure that cake is essential to the subject though always nice to have. Finity UK[5] has produced a guide for people who want to run workshops about dying, death and loss within their own community.

Our chapter 12: *Practical Matters* gave information on writing a Will and preparing a Power of Attorney, and chapter 3: *Difficult Decisions* spoke about an Advanced Decision document.

What can we say and do when friends or family have some bad news and are facing the possibility or even probability of an earlier death than they ever anticipated?

> 'Talking about death at the end of life is a difficult, awkward proposition for both the dying person and for family members. Each may have different reasons for wanting to stay silent or to talk. Some family members say nothing, out of fear of saying the wrong thing. Or the dying person says nothing because of a superstitious belief that to acknowledge death is to hasten it. And family members often want to shield their grief from the dying person, while the dying person similarly wants to protect family members. I wanted to talk to her about death, but there was always this feeling of hope that she was going to make it.'
>
> Words of a son whose mother died without a conversation about dying.[6]

The main thing about talking to a person who is facing the possibility of a shortened life span, or someone close to them who is going to be affected by their illness or death, is *listening*.

Initially, after a life-threatening diagnosis the person

can be numb with shock. If you are involved at this time you can probably do little else but sit with them showing that you care. Holding a hand can be a powerful means of communication. If you are there, sitting silently, and they want to talk, they will do so.

> 'Communication is what human beings do, even if it's just holding someone's hand.'
>
> Dr S J. Baumrucker, associate editor in chief of the
> *American Journal of Hospice and Palliative Care.*[7]

If you are a close friend or family and have indicated that you care, you might need to listen over and over again, to the same story. This process can be very important and patience is needed.

If you are like those quoted above, not wanting to make things worse by talking about the illness you can be sure that almost always the person will find some relief in being able to talk about what is surely on their mind.

Making a comment such as: 'This must be very difficult for you', or maybe a question: 'Do you want to talk about it?' is usually the way in. You might be rejected – if so, 'back off'. Nothing will have been lost. There is a lot more to be lost by not giving the opportunity for a conversation that is needed.

> 'Walking in the alien land of illness that few friends and relatives know how to enter, some days I am eager to talk about my feelings about the illness and treatment, on others I am just tired of thinking about my illness at all, I never know what mood I will be in but I would be delighted to have my friends ask bluntly what I feel like talking about.'
>
> Elizabeth Burnham[8]

You might not be a close friend or relative, but people do not always open up to those close to them. It can be a relief to find someone willing to listen, to help them get things sorted in their own mind. You don't need to 'fix' it for them, just listen unless or until you are asked a question.

It is important to know that sometimes when you are trying to help there is anger at the situation and if this is directed at you (because you happen to be in the firing line) do your utmost not to retaliate but soak it up – though it may seem so, it is not, in fact, personal.

We need to talk, communicate, share feelings and cry together.

> 'When I first went to Burrswood, when people cried, I used to over-comfort them out of my own need. When they were crying I might put a hand out and say, 'It's all right' and stem the flow. That isn't always helpful. We need to cry and sometimes tears are part of our healing. Count it as a privilege when people feel safe enough with you to cry.'
>
> Gareth Tuckwell

What is important in the dying phase?

To understand that death is near

People do need to know from the doctors that they are nearing death. As a cancer doctor I (ES) often thought it must be obvious to the patient and family when things were not good and that death sooner rather than later was inevitable. Often this was not the case. They did not have my experience. Unless the doctor pronounced, they thought there was no need to worry, life was secure and probably more treatment would be available. However just *when* death will occur is not possible to say and life can be considerably shorter or longer than any doctor predicts.

'Doctors are still not good at talking about dying. Less than half of the patients who were capable of understanding were told that they were dying. Only a fifth were asked about spiritual needs. How can we involve patients in decision-making if we don't tell them what is happening? How can they make their spiritual or cultural preparations if they don't know what they are facing? How can we treat people according to their beliefs and wishes if we do not ask them what they are?'

Dr David Brooks,
Past President of the Association for Palliative Medicine of GB and Ireland [9]

Only a fifth of patients in the National Care of the Dying Audit England 2014 [10] were asked about spiritual needs, which can be explained as a person's deepest relationships: with others, themselves and with God.

Spiritual as well as physical needs

'Dying is more than a physical event. Rather, the experience reaches us on all levels — psychological, social, and of course, spiritual. We cannot neglect the spiritual needs any more than we can neglect the physical needs. Care for the dying is inherently holistic.' [11]

Those approaching death in old age have been found to want to look back over their lives, to reminisce, look at photos and perhaps revisit favourite places.

They want to die in a way that is consistent with their values, wishes and earlier life.

They want to find hope beyond the grave.

'One minister has confessed: 'We talk a lot about what we believe comes after death. But we skip pretty quickly over dying itself, except to say, "Make your peace with the Lord." Doubts and questions can be taken as a sign of a weak faith. As a result, Christians can still find that their faith gives them no guidance about how to live the final chapter of life.'

Spiritual Issues at the End of Life
John Hardwick, Professor of Philosophy[12]

Family

This is the time to encourage attempts to reconcile family members and resolve family disagreements – before it is too late.

'After family members are dead is not a good time to try to reconcile with them.'[13]

When people first realise they have a life-shortening illness they often want to take care of family members. Then as death draws closer they become more introspective, and this is often the opportunity for meaningful discussion. You can ask: 'How do you think you are doing just now?' If the answer is 'Not so well', the person is looking for a chance to talk. Try to ask: 'Do you want to talk about it?'

Those who work in the field of death and dying emphasise that acknowledging the end of life and saying goodbye, in whatever form, is an emotional and even a physical balm, reducing stress and depression.

Hospice workers find that, as death approaches, words become less important, touch and silence become more meaningful. Music, for some families, has its own language.

A niece had tried to talk to her aunt about the differences they'd had and was rebuffed. Finally, she had the conversation she'd wanted by singing Amazing Grace to her aunt, who lay in bed, close to death. 'I wasn't sure I could do it, but I did,' she says. 'I felt she could hear me. She squeezed my hand.'[14]

Acceptance of Loss

'People facing death suffer from an inability to find meaning in this last chapter of their lives; from a bleak, narrowly confined and abbreviated future; from inability to deal meaningfully with family and loved ones at this final opportunity – from total dependence on others; from loss of capabilities; from being turned from a contributor into a burden on others; from the indignity of being unable to take care of even basic bodily functions; from a sense that their bodies or their minds are betraying them; from being cast out of the world in which the healthy live; from guilt; from a sense of abandonment; from anger about all of this; *and from isolation due to the reluctance of the healthy to broach the subject of dying.*

'I submit that patient and family issues at the end of life are almost entirely *spiritual*, for perhaps especially at the end of life, we become aware that we are spiritual beings.'

John Hardwick[15]

Can we encourage those living into a frail old age to consider how they want to live before they die and even how they want to die?

Purposeful living

There are challenges here for family, medical, nursing and care home staff. Atul Gawande, in his book *Being Mortal*,[16] urges us to give the elderly more independence, allow them to take risks, incorporate children and animals into their lives and generally give life a purpose other than waiting in safety to die. These ideas are being taken up in some nursing and care homes.

The elderly could, as a matter of course, be encouraged to talk about their aims and wishes for their remaining days, months or years as well as where and how they wish to die. (See chapter 4: *Talking about dying: when, where and how?*)

This last phase of life will be a challenge. Can it also be an opportunity?

Prayer?

For those who believe in a loving and caring God, prayer is valued, but let the person know that you are praying.

Those who are grieving for loss of health or in bereavement often say they cannot pray; it is important that others take on that 'job' for them.

'Prayer for a person in need is something in which we can all participate. When we pray for people we stand before God as their representative.'

Elizabeth Heike, *A Question of Grief* [17]

If you are a person of faith it might be appropriate to ask the person if they would like prayer. If you pray, keep it short and simple. Christians have found familiar prayers (e.g. the Lord's Prayer; the Evening Collect or J. H. Newman's *O Lord support us all the day long*) to be helpful – but sensitivity to the person is crucial.

O Lord, support us
all the day long,
until the shadows lengthen,
and the evening comes,
and the busy world is hushed,
and the fever of life is over,
and our work is done.

Then in your mercy,
grant us a safe lodging and a holy rest,
and peace at the last.

Amen.

Death as a release

The event of death can be a relief for a spouse or parent who has already been grieving in anticipation.

> After the death of my cousin aged 45 from oesophageal cancer my aunt wrote to me in India: 'It's all over for Jeffrey now, no more pain and suffering.'   (ES)

On the other hand, for one who has devoted themselves to caring there is always a deeply lonely existence when the one who has consumed time, energy and thought is no longer there.

My father was devastated when my mother with Alzheimer's-type dementia went into a home rather against his will, although she was getting too difficult for him to handle and keep safe. He exchanged the frustration of the changes that had taken place and the difficulties of caring for the wife who had looked after him for over 30 years, for the dreadful loneliness of being at home on his own.

End Piece

We trust that this book will be both an encouragement and a source of hope. Where is this hope to come from? For us and for many, it comes from our Christian faith that God does not want death to be the end for us but only the gateway to everlasting life. And he sent Jesus to overcome death and sin for us – and he showed that he had done this by rising from the dead. We can be confident of this because the Bible's New Testament reports the evidence of his meeting, not only with his special friends, the apostles, but with hundreds of other people as well.

One of those was a man on a journey to Damascus all fired up to arrest and kill Christian believers. That man was Paul who after his dramatic conversion wrote those powerful words of confident hope which we quoted at the end of chapter one. It is worth pondering them and sharing them as we grapple with the challenges that dying brings. We do not need to face it alone for, in spite of all the agonies, physical and emotional, death may bring, the love of Jesus Christ Himself will be with us.

As St Paul said:

I am convinced that neither death nor life . . . neither the present nor the future, nor any powers, neither height nor depth or anything else in all creation, will be able to separate us from the love of God that is in Christ Jesus our Lord (Romans 8:38-39).

That is why, whether we are the person dying or we are facing the death of someone close to us, we can and should talk about dying with confidence and hope. Had I [PG] had a book like this available when Duncan telephoned me, it would have been so much easier to talk to him and his wife about preparing for his death.

Notes

[1] Liberating the NHS DH 2012

[2] Ellen Goodman (*New York Times*) speaking to friends about family deaths http://opinionator.blogs.nytimes.com/2015/07/01/how-to-talk-about-dying/?_r=0

[3] deathcafes.com

[4] https://churchofenglandfunerals.org/gravetalk

[5] www.finity.org.uk

[6] WebMD URAC accredited health information website: www.webmd.com/healthy-aging/features/talk-about-death

[7] Dr S. J. Baumrucker, associate editor in chief of the *American Journal of Hospice and Palliative Care* : www.webmd.com/healthy-aging/features/talk-about-death

[8] Elizabeth Burnham, Elizabeth, *When your Friend is Dying* (Kingsway, 1982), p24.

[9] Dr David Brooks past president of the Association for Palliative Medicine of GB and Ireland in *The Guardian*, reporting on the National care of the dying audit for hospitals in England May 2014: www.theguardian.com/commentisfree/2014/may/15/doctors-talking-about-dying-patients-palliative-care

[10] www.rcplondon.ac.uk/projects/outputs/national-care-dying-audit-hospitals

[11] Adapted from: *Living with Grief: Spirituality and End-of-Life Care*, ed., Kenneth J Doka, Amy S. Tucci, and Keith G Meador, Hospice Foundation of America, 2011.

[12] http://web.utk.edu/~jhardwig/spiritua.htm

[13] Baumrucker, see Note 7.

[14] Jane Meredith Adams in WebMD:
www.webmd.com/healthy-aging/features/talk-about-death

[15] 'Spiritual Issues at the End of Life', John Hardwick, Professor of Philosophy. See Note 12.

[16] Profile Books, London (2014)

[17] Hodder and Stoughton, 1985, pp.116-117

APPENDIX 1

PREPARING FOR AN EXPECTED DEATH AT HOME

Elaine Sugden

In our experience, many people with an imminently terminal illness want to die at home where they feel safe and comfortable. However, for the family facing the death of a close friend or relative at home can be a time of ongoing worry.

To die at home is often a last wish. Loving carers are needed to make this happen and though professional carers are available they are unlikely to be so 24 hours a day. Family and friend carers are still needed and will probably be preferred by the one dying. Most homes, though not all, are suitable for the death of a frail person needing personal help.

Local doctors and nurses can provide the necessary equipment as well as expert pain and other symptom relief, but a lot of responsibility falls on close family and friends. Contemplating managing a death at home requires thought, a quiet determination and a small band of practical and acceptable helpers. It might not be easy but can be a final act of love and devotion.

Few of us have witnessed a death. What exactly is going to happen and how will we cope? When I was working as a cancer doctor I was often asked 'what will happen?' My answer in general was that the person would become weaker and at the end gradually fade away. Now, having become involved with friends in my community whose close relatives have died or are expected to die in the near future, I realise that this, though generally true, was an inadequate explanation. Faced with this situation we need to know more.

The most frequent questions are:

When will it happen?
How will I know it is happening?
What will happen?

When will death happen? The medical team prepares and gives as much information as possible. They make sure appropriate and sufficient medication is available. But no one can be sure just when death will occur. Doctors and nurses can only give an estimate and are often surprised themselves by how long or how short a time someone in this situation lives.

How will I know and what will happen? These questions have a similar answer and we have listed the indications that the end is coming as the body gradually shuts down and prepares for the end of life:

Eating and drinking often becomes less and chewing and swallowing slower. Small amounts especially of what is fancied should be offered but not forced. Dry lips can be moistened.

Quietness is often preferred as is the presence of just a few or even only one person. With weakness and tiredness speech is often slow or even impossible.

Sleeping usually increases, communication decreases and at times the person might become unresponsive or not able to be roused. This is a time to sit with them, holding their hand and speaking softly. They are likely to continue be able to hear even if they seem to be asleep.

Restlessness can occur with the bodily changes. Try not to fight this but speak calmly and reassuringly. Light hand or forehead massage, reading or playing soft music sometimes helps.

Disorientation or confusion can occur.
Try not to contradict what the person is saying. Listen respectfully. Not infrequently the dying person 'sees' people who died some time ago or 'sees' angels appearing in the room or at the window. These are not hallucinations or anything to do with the medication but the 'normal' detachment from this life.

Other changes as death approaches.
Incontinence of bladder and bowels can occur so that effective pads and bed protection are needed. The District Nurse might be able to supply these 'just in case'. The urine can become very concentrated and look like strong tea. This happens as the kidneys gradually shut down.

Changes in breathing: fast, slow or with gaps can occur. Unusual breathing noises are common and the skin colour can change and become dusky. If the arms and legs feel cold try using covers but be prepared for the person to throw them off. A light sheet might be tolerated. These are all normal changes and do not need to produce alarm. These changes are not easy for those caring to experience but the care and presence of the family or close friends is an act of great love, which you can give at the end of life.

Saying goodbye can be an important part of dying. Often the dying person wants to see those who have been special to them over the years. They might 'hang on' until they have seen those they need to and until they can be sure that those left behind will be OK without them. Family and friends need to be able to confirm that they will be OK and give 'permission' for the person to leave. Tears are normal and do not need to be hidden.

At the time of death breathing and heartbeats stop, the person relaxes so that the eyes are partially open, the jaw slack and sometimes the bladder and/or bowel empty.

This is a time to be still or, if you are alone, to call someone to be with you. It might be appropriate for the family to have discussed, at an earlier time, who will be called and when.

There is no urgency to call the doctor or funeral director. This can be done all in good time. Death often occurs during the night and if so it is reasonable, as long as a friend or relative is with you, to wait until the GP surgery opens in the morning to report the death.

February 2016

Sources:

www.caregiverslibrary.org/caregivers-resources/grp-end-of-life-issues/preparing-for-the-death-of-a-loved-one-article.aspx

www.cancerresearchuk.org/about-cancer/coping-with-cancer/dying/decisions/choosing-where-to-die

APPENDIX 2

MORE PRACTICAL HELP

Philip Giddings and Elaine Sugden

- **Practical help relevant to all these situations**

Specific help

We need to offer specific help. It is best not to say 'Let me know if I can help' because this rarely happens. However, if you are the one with the difficult diagnosis or the one bereaved, please be prepared to ask for, or agree to, an offer of help. Your family and friends are likely to be desperate to share in some way in your suffering and you will be helping them as much as they are helping you.

There are many possibilities for help depending on your own particular gifts, experiences and abilities as well as the particular circumstances:

Invitations out, delivered meals (food in disposable containers helps) transport, washing and ironing, cleaning, gardening, help with correspondence, reading aloud, small household maintenance jobs, etc. Ask what would help and offer what you can do.

Leaving people alone is not usually the best thing to do unless they have requested this. Let them know you care and later on that you still care, however much time has gone by. Often friendship, help and understanding are needed for much longer than we think. Offer your own particular skills – and we must all learn to listen.

Short times are best, especially if the person does not know you well. Even those who were 'get up and go' people can experience inertia, and jobs get left undone – having someone to do them can be helpful. Offers might need to be specific: 'Can I come around this week and do a few jobs for you?' Or perhaps: 'I am coming round, please find a job for me to do.' Some jobs for the bereaved will be full of memories and help might not be welcome; try to be sensitive.

But be flexible, the answer might be 'not needed just now' – be conscious that the person or family might need time alone.

Phone calls, e-mails and letters might be appreciated. Visits should be offered rather than just turning up and, if necessary, it is best to have arranged somewhere to stay other than with the person or their family. Go with a purpose, not out of guilt or obligation. Check whether taking anything would be appropriate – it is possible to have a surfeit of flowers/grapes/chocolate.

The limits of help

Support your friends and family simply as friends or family and with common sense. Remember you are not a trained counsellor and sometimes professional help from a GP or a counsellor will be needed. For information, see NHS choices: counselling (website details at (C) below).

Look after yourself

You as a friend will need other friends to share concerns and experiences with. A small network of people offering support to the sufferer as well as to one another can work well.

• In Bereavement

For those wishing to help but who have not experienced significant bereavement themselves there are some things to be aware of:

It is different for everyone
Whatever the timing or situation of death the bereaved individual's experience of and response to loss is different. It is impossible for those who have not been through the death of someone emotionally close to know how bereavement feels.

It is a long up and down process
Bereavement is a long, often 'roller coaster' process. Just when you think you are coming out of it you are overwhelmed again. It is not something that can be 'snapped out of' – everyone needs to go at their own speed and should not compare themselves with others.

The cycle of the year is important. Christmas and birthdays are often difficult times, as can be family and other gatherings when the significant someone is missing. The death anniversary is a particularly difficult time. Weekends and winter evenings can seem endless, lonely times.

For some, several years might go by before the promised 'it will get better' eventually comes. The special someone will never be forgotten but a 'new normal' is established and life can go on.

'This will be my second Christmas without Shelley, and I think of her every day. It's not so much that the hurt and empty void disappear, more that you learn to live with it, and remember the good times. I can still hear her laughter echoing down the hallway and she will always be with me.'   David, a young widower

---

Does anything help?

Some benefit from activity – having a programme of things that must be done. Those who have children to care for don't have much choice; they must carry on. Exercise is important and can be helpful; it might be a way of meeting people.

The most unexpected people are especially helpful and seem to know what you need. Others of your friends might find it difficult to understand.

It is said that those with faith in general fare better. But even if you are a true believer that death is not the end, there remains the 'Dark Night' of the soul.

Letter and cards are appreciated, especially if they speak about the one who has died and avoid platitudes such as 'a happy release' or 'a good death' which can be upsetting to the one left in bereavement.

'Some of our friends and family still mark the anniversary of C's death by giving us flowers, or sending a card: this is much appreciated.'

A father several years after his daughter's death as a young adult.

Talk about the one who has died. Listen, don't jump in with suggestions. Let the bereaved talk about what they want to talk about. There might be anger: at God, at the person who has 'left' them, at others who haven't shown appropriate care or understanding. There might be tears, guilt, and always a deep, deep sadness. Don't be frightened of tears. Weep with those who weep. Only in heaven will there be no more tears.

Eating alone is hard; hospitality provides company as well as food.

'We (the bereaved) may find that we have changed from a self-confident decisive person into an uncertain confused and procrastinating individual. As time went on I discovered a child within myself who wanted, and at times I believe needed, someone to take responsibilities from me, make decisions and generally relieve me of the burden of keeping the wheels of my own life turning.'

Elizabeth Heike, *A Question of Grief*
Hodder and Stoughton, 1985, p73

Keep on remembering

'It is still helpful and nice to hear others' memories of the person. Don't think we won't be interested or will break down or be upset.'

Mother of 19-year-old who died by suicide several years ago.

'We would have liked more opportunity, in the years after C died and up to the present, to talk to others about her, e.g. to say how proud we were of her strengths and achievements. We would be hesitant to start such a conversation, not wanting to be thought to be looking backwards. No doubt some friends, who knew C, and even family, think it might upset us to talk about her, but the opposite is true.'

C's parents, several years after their daughter's death as a young adult.

• **Other helpful resources**

Burnham, Elizabeth, *When your Friend is Dying* (Kingsway, 1982).

Fawcett, Nick, *Living with Loss: Poems to Inspire Prayer*, (Kevin Mayhew Ltd, 2005).

NHS choices, counselling: http://www.nhs.uk/conditions/Counselling/Pages/Introduction.aspx

From the New Testament: Romans 8:38-39

• **Prayers which may be helpful**

The Third Collect at Evening Prayer
(*Book of Common Prayer*)

Lighten our darkness, we beseech thee, O Lord;
and by thy great mercy defend us from all perils and
dangers of this night;
for the love of thy only Son, our Saviour Jesus Christ.
Amen.

J. H. Newman: *Lead, Kindly Light*

Lead, Kindly Light, amidst th'encircling gloom,
Lead Thou me on!
The night is dark, and I am far from home,
Lead Thou me on!
Keep Thou my feet; I do not ask to see
The distant scene; one step enough for me.

I was not ever thus, nor prayed that Thou
Shouldst lead me on;
I loved to choose and see my path; but now
Lead Thou me on!
I loved the garish day, and, spite of fears,
Pride ruled my will. Remember not past years!

So long Thy power hath blest me, sure it still
Will lead me on.
O'er moor and fen, o'er crag and torrent, till
The night is gone,
And with the morn those angel faces smile,
Which I have loved long since, and lost awhile!

Meantime, along the narrow rugged path,
Thyself hast trod,
Lead, Saviour, lead me home in childlike faith,
Home to my God.
To rest forever after earthly strife
In the calm light of everlasting life.

The Lord's Prayer (Church of England, *Common Worship*)

Our Father in heaven,
hallowed be your name.
Your Kingdom come,
your will be done,
on earth as in heaven.
Give us today our daily bread.
Forgive us our sins
as we forgive those who sin against us.
Lead us not into temptation
but deliver us from evil.
For the kingdom,
the power, and the glory are yours
now and for ever.

Amen.

The Lord's Prayer (*Book of Common Prayer*)

Our Father which art in heaven,
Hallowed be thy Name,
Thy kingdom come,
Thy will be done,
in earth as it is in heaven.
Give us this day our daily bread;
And forgive us our trespasses,
As we forgive them that trespass against us;
And lead us not into temptation,
But deliver us from evil.
For thine is the kingdom,
the power, and the glory,
For ever and ever.

Amen.

APPENDIX 3

Advanced Directive/Advanced Decision (Living Will)

Elaine Sugden

Medical science has made enormous strides in the past 50-60 years. Diseases and conditions that previously meant almost certain death can now be cured or held at bay. Many people are living into their eighties and nineties with a good quality of life, although inevitably with increasing frailty. This is of course very good.

However, sometimes the body can be 'kept going' even when quality of life, in spite of all medical efforts, is very poor. Doctors themselves find it difficult to know whether or not to keep on trying to keep a patient, who is not fully conscious, alive. He or she can be put onto a ventilator (breathing machine) or provided with a feeding tube. The age, frailty and likelihood of improvement of each person need to be considered. An elderly patient whose heart stops working can have attempted resuscitation, but this is unlikely to be successful and makes their last moments anything but peaceful. In my experience when doctors are unsure, they will almost always do something to keep the person alive.

For these reasons those who want to be involved in decisions about their own medical care at the end of life can sign (before a witness) what is commonly known as a Living Will. This is more correctly known in Scotland as an Advanced Directive and in England as an Advanced Decision. Both are covered by the abbreviation: AD.

Most of the websites below give more information about the medical situations where an AD might be useful.

The document I recently filled in for myself has questions about what I want to do if:

I have a terminal illness that is nearing the end of its course;
I am unconscious and unlikely to regain consciousness;
I am severely and permanently mentally impaired.

I have written that in all these cases I do not want to be resuscitated if my heart stops, I do not want to be tube fed and I do not want to be put onto a breathing machine.

You might answer the questions differently; there are no right or wrong answers, just your answers. It is good to think about and discuss these possible situations.

After signing, copies can be given to those you wish – relatives, special friends and your doctor. The signed document is legally binding, but if you are unconscious or severely mentally impaired, someone else has to inform the medical staff of your wishes.

Every year or so, check to see if your wishes have changed; if they have, you might need a new document. If your answers would not change, sign the document again with the new date on the document. If there are any changes let your family, friends and doctor know.

Useful Websites

Age UK
www.ageuk.org.uk/documents/en-gb/factsheets/fs72_advance_decisions_advance_statements_and_living_wills_fcs.pdf?dtrk=true

Alzheimer's society
www.alzheimers.org.uk/site/scripts/documents_info.php?documentID=143

Compassion in dying
http://compassionindying.org.uk/making-decisions-and-planning-your-care/ has downloadable forms in normal and large print to download and fill in.

Dying Matters
http://dyingmatters.org/page/planning-ahead

LawDepot provides forms to fill in with your wishes but not a lot of information
www.lawdepot.co.uk/contracts/living-will-advance-directive/?loc=GB&pid=googleppc-health_uk-WillT1_e2-s-ggkey_advanced%20decisions&s_kwcid=advanced%20decisions|60245949383&gclid=CJv5sM6YkMkCFUHlwgodl84CYg

Macmillan
www.macmillan.org.uk/Cancerinformation/Livingwithandaftercancer/Advancedcancer/AdvanceDecision.aspx

NHS choices has links to other helpful web sites.
www.nhs.uk/Planners/end-of-life-care/Pages/advance-decision-to-refuse-treatment.aspx

February 2016

BIBLIOGRAPHY

Burnham, Elizabeth Dean, *When your Friend is Dying* (Kingsway Publications, 1983)

Craig, William Lane, *The Son Rises* (Wipf and Stock, 2000)

Dominica, Sister Frances, Just My Reflection – helping parents do things their way when their child dies, www.helen&douglas house org.uk

Doka, Kenneth J, Tucci, Amy S. and Meador, Keith G (Eds.), *Living with Grief: Spirituality and End-of-Life Care*, (Hospice Foundation of America, 2011)

Down, Martin *The Christian Hope: a Guide to Life after Death* (Rehoboth Media, 2016)

Drain, Andrew J, *Code Red* (Christian Medical Fellowship, 2010)

Gawande, Atul, *Being Mortal* (Pro le Books, Wellcome Collection, 2014)

Graham, Billy, *Nearing Home, Life, Faith and Finishing Well* (Thomas Nelson, 2011)

Habermas, Gary *The Case for the Resurrection of Jesus* (Kregel Publications, 2004)

Heike, Elizabeth, *A Question of Grief* Hodder and Stoughton, 1985

Levine, Stephen, *Who Dies: An Investigation of Conscious Living and Conscious Dying*, (Gateway Books)

McQuellon, Richard P, and Cowan, Michael A, *The Art of Conversation through Serious Illness* (Oxford University Press, 2010)

Moltmann, Jürgen, *God in Creation*, Fortress Publishing, 1993

Morrison, Frank, *Who Moved the Stone?* (Authentic Media)

Spufford, Margaret, *Celebration* (Continuum International Publishing, 1996)

Twycross, Robert *A Time to Die* (Christian Medical Fellowship, 1994)

Wertheimer, Alison *A Special Scar – The Experiences of People Bereaved by Suicide* (Routledge, 1992)

Worth, Jennifer, *In the Midst of Life* (Weidenfeld & Nicolson, 2012)

Wright, Tom *Surprised by Hope* (SPCK, 2011)

Facing the death of your child, Children's Cancer and Leukaemia Group CCLG publications, April 2015

As Big as it Gets: supporting a child when a parent is seriously ill, Winston's Wish 2012

Beyond the Rough Rock: supporting a child who has been bereaved through suicide, Winston's Wish 2008

What Happens When Someone Dies: A book for adults and children to share together (SeeSaw publication 2014)

ADDITIONAL WEBSITES

Alzheimer's Society: www.alzheimers.org.uk
Arranging a funeral: www.gov.uk/after-a-death/arrange-the-funeral
Babycentre general: www.babycentre.co.uk
Babyloss: www.babyloss.com/index.php
Care for the family bereaved parent support:
www.careforthefamily.org.uk/bps
Care for the Family widowed young support:
www.careforthefamily.org.uk/wys
Citizens Advice Bureau:
www.citizensadvice.org.uk/relationships/death-and-wills
Child Bereavement UK: http://childbereavementuk.org
Death Cafes: http://deathcafe.com
Dying Matters: http://www.dyingmatters.org
Grave Talk: https://churchofenglandfunerals.org/gravetalk
Living with Dying (healthtalk.org):
www.healthtalk.org/peoples-experiences/dying-bereavement/living-dying/topics
Lullaby Trust: www.lullabytrust.org.uk
Lasting Power of Attorney:
www.gov.uk/power-of-attorney/overview
Macmillan Cancer support: www.macmillan.org.uk
Making a Will:
www.gov.uk/make-will/overview
www.lawsociety.org.uk/for-the-public/common-legal-issues/making-a-will
Marie Curie Cancer Care: www.mariecurie.org.uk
Miscarriage Association (MA): www.miscarriageassociation.org.uk
National Association of Funeral Directors:
www.nafd.org.uk/funeral-advice/find-a-member
The National Society Of Allied And Independent Funeral Directors: http://saif.org.uk/members-search
National Council for Palliative Care: www.ncpc.org.uk
National Institute for Health and Care Excellence (NICE):
www.nice.org.uk
NHS Advanced Care Planning and Advanced Directives:
www.nhs.uk/Planners/end-of-life-care/Pages/planning-ahead.aspx
Office of National Statistics (ONS): http://ons.gov.uk

Organ Donation:
www.organdonation.nhs.uk/register-to-donate
Preparing for a death:
www.caregiverslibrary.org/caregivers-resources/grp-end-of-life-issues/
preparing-for-the-death-of-a-loved-one-article.aspx
www.cancerresearchuk.org/about-cancer/coping-with-cancer/dying/
decisions/choosing-where-to-die
Resuscitation Council (UK): www.resus.org.uk
Samaritans website: www.samaritans.org
SANDS Stillbirth and neonatal death charity: www.uk-sands.org
Together for Short Lives: www.togetherforshortlives.org.uk
WebMD talk about death:
www.webmd.com/healthy-aging/features/talk-about-death
What to do when someone dies:
1. www.gov.uk/after-a-death/overview
2. www.nhs.uk/ipgmedia/national/lymphoma%20association/assets/
whattodowhensomeonedies(la8pages).pdf
Winston's Wish: www.winstonswish.org.uk

ABOUT THE AUTHORS

Philip Giddings taught at the University of Reading from 1972 until his retirement as Head of the School of Politics and International Relations in 2011. An elected member of the Church of England's General Synod from 1985 to 2015 and of Archbishops' Council from 2001 to 2015, he chaired its Mission and Public Affairs Council from 2003 to 2011. He has twice been widowed. His other publications are in the field of Parliamentary affairs and the Ombudsman institution.

Martin Down is an Anglican priest who served in country parishes in Lincolnshire and Norfolk until 2012 when he retired to live in Oxfordshire. He is the author of several other books including *The Best Is Yet To Be: Being happy in retirement and old age*, and *The Christian Hope: A guide to life after death*.

Elaine Sugden worked in Leeds as a doctor of children with leukaemia in the 1970s before moving with her family to India for 6 years. Since 1984 she worked in adult oncology in Oxford, from 1995 as a consultant treating adults and children with cancer. She retired in 2013 but continues to be involved in a European organisation working for those treated for cancer as children. Her booklet *Caring for People with Cancer*, based on a series of seminars in India, was published in 1998.

Gareth Tuckwell was Medical Director of Burrswood Christian Hospital and then CEO between 1986-2012. He has been involved with Macmillan Cancer Support as both a regional director and trustee. Clinical Director of Hospice in the Weald from 2003-2007, he is vice-president of Phyllis Tuckwell Hospice Care. He currently chairs Sanctuary Care which provides residential care to 3500 people and the M.E. Trust for myalgic encephalomyelitis which provides treatment and care for people with M.E.

Gareth contributed to 'A Time to Heal', a report for The House of Bishops in 2000, *A Question of Healing* (Eagle, 2000), 'Transforming Health' (MARC, 2005) and 'Mud and Stars' (1991) the report on the impact of hospice experience on the Church's understanding of healing.

Printed in Great Britain
by Amazon